# Humor
# and the Health
# Professions
## The Therapeutic Use of Humor in Health Care

## Second Edition

## Vera M. Robinson, EdD, RN
Professor Emeritus
Department of Nursing
California State University
Fullerton, California

**SLACK** Incorporated
6900 Grove Road
Thorofare, NJ

Executive Editor:   Cheryl D. Willoughby
Publisher:   Harry C. Benson

Printed in the United States of America

Library of Congress Catalog Card Number: 89-043106

ISBN: 1-55642-141-9

Published by:  SLACK Incorporated
               6900 Grove Road
               Thorofare, NJ 08086-9447

Last digit is print number:   10   9   8   7   6   5   4   3   2

# Dedication

To all the many colleagues, friends, students, and patients who have shared their humor, their laughter, their knowledge, and their expertise—with gratitude, love, and laughter.

# Contents

# Preface

## Second Edition

Since the first publication of this book, which was a pioneering effort in applying the concept of humor to health care, there has been a major change in the acceptance, recognition and utilization of humor. Humor is "in"!

We have moved from a time when humor was not considered a "scholarly" subject to investigate, and when laughter in health care was not encouraged or sanctioned by the system. We have progressed from humor as a "light topic" luncheon speaker, to keynoting major conferences, presenting workshops, and serving as consultant and resource for graduate students, researchers, health care agencies, lay groups, and individuals seeking the "healing power" of humor.

There has been a proliferation of studies, research and education on humor since I completed the original research in this book. The numbers of published articles and books in all areas of humor has multiplied at an astonishing rate. There is a "humor movement" that has reached into all segments of society! No longer considered "trivial," humor is recognized as an important ingredient in life, and in mental and physical health.

What has contributed to this surge of interest and acceptance? One of the major factors has been the increased stresses of living in today's world and the accompanying movement toward health promotion, wellness and self-care. Society has become concerned with prevention and healthy behaviors: the reduction and management of stress, good nutrition, exercise, a healthy lifestyle, and a positive attitude toward life. Similarly, in the health care field, we have moved from a disease orientation to a focus on health promotion in our practice. Positive behaviors and positive emotions, self-care, holistic health, hope, love, play, laughter and caring have become accepted practice and a basis for scholarly study.

Perhaps the catalyst for the movement of humor and health was the report in 1977 of Norman Cousins who, through programmed sessions of laughter, recovered from ankylosing spondilitis, a life-threatening disease (1979). Suddenly, the work of major humor researchers begun in the late 60's and early 70's, was recognized. It spurred more study into the origin and development of humor; the physiology of laughter; the psychology and sociology of humor; humor and education; and humor and health. Studies have broadened to include ways to increase the humorous outlook; humor and stress, humor in the workplace; humor and culture; humor in psychotherapy; in aging, and with children, and in care of the terminally ill. Major research continues on laughter's effect on the immune system and the biochemical effects of all the positive emotions.

At the same time, the Workshop Library on World Humor was born in Washington, D.C in 1975. Its purpose was to encourage and explore the uses of humor and collect and examine the world's humor heritage. In 1976, the group held the First International Conference on Humor in Cardiff, Wales. The Seventh International Conference on Humor was held in Hawaii in 1989. Out of these meetings of scholars was formed the International Journal of Humor Research and the International Society for Humor Studies was organized in 1989.

In the interim years, many other groups, organizations and projects have been formed to promote humor, sponsor meetings, workshops and conferences. Humor "specialists" in every field have emerged, offering education on the use of humor, play, and laughter to the general public, to industry, management, educators and health care groups. Newsletters, magazines, humor materials, joke books and joke lines have surfaced. Articles on the value and beneficial effects of humor and laughter have appeared in popular as well as professional magazines.

Although controversy over the use of humor and its beneficial effects continues within the academic and professional community, and, much more empirical evidence is still needed, humor and laughter have become acclaimed as healthy and healing tools to reduce stress, promote health, aid in illness and suffering, and, in general, increase the quality of life. Humor has become a serious business!

In the health care field, the need for understanding humor and increasing one's skill in application has taken on major proportions.

The foundation presented in the first edition of this book is still viable and applicable. This basic research was begun in 1965, the same time others were looking at the grief process, at the concept of love, hope, and other positive emotions. It was a time when the methodology for grounded theory and qualitative research was not yet well defined or well received in scientific circles. Yet the application of humor to health and health care required this approach. Basic questions needed to be answered. What was the nature of humor as it occurred in this setting? Why did it occur? And, how could we cultivate its use as a therapeutic tool? My research identified the functions, purposes and application of humor in health care, utilizing observations from the setting and the theories, research and literature from the natural and behavioral sciences as well as the humanities.

This second edition will add to this base and incorporate the new research and studies from the past decade, including my own continuing research in the use of humor in health care.

It will expand on the communication, social, and psycho-logical functions of humor, on the physiological and biochemical effects on the body and the mind-body interaction. It will extend the benefits of laughter to the health professional in preventing burnout and in management. More specifics related to patient education, to use with children, the elderly, and in various clinical areas will be included.

The guidelines for cultivating and increasing one's humorous attitude and skills in applying and utilizing humor as a therapeutic intervention with clients, colleagues, students, and others also will be expanded.

There will be many more humorous anecdotes and examples of humorous strategies and techniques, as well as canned humor and those spontaneous, unintentional laughable incidents that occur daily in health care. We hope these will aid in your understanding of the therapeutic role of humor, and will also stimulate your own "sense of humor," spark your creativity, and allow your own inherent capacity for comedy and for humorous interaction to emerge.

> "If we consider the frequent reliefs we receive from laughter, and how often it breaks the gloom which is apt to depress the mind, one would take care not to grow too wise for so great a pleasure of life." Joseph Addison

# Preface

## First Edition

Humor is a form of communication highly regarded in our society. As the vast amount of literature can attest, there has always been a need for laughter and comedy. Humor has been described as a pleasure upon which man pounces at the slightest excuse to indulge in it. No one denies its value. It is a part of our lives even in times of stress, danger, and death. Yet, despite our recognition of its value, we do not take humor seriously. We are afraid to look at and analyze humor — to make conscious, deliberate use of humor as a tool in communication and as a way of intervening in the stresses of living. We allow it to happen by chance. There has been little or no attempt at a planned use of humor, particularly in the health professions.

The time is ripe for health professionals to do more than just enjoy humor. We need to understand it. We need to be able to laugh at ourselves, at life and at our establishments. We need to begin to help our students and patients to deal with their stresses, tensions and frustrations through the use of humor. We need to believe that humor is constructive and healthy; we must encourage its use as a coping mechanism, and cultivate its use as a viable tool in communication.

The aim of this study is to go beyond the description of humor and theorizing about its nature — the primary focus of other authors and researchers — and to provide some beginning guidelines for cultivating the concept of humor as a planned tool in teaching, in communication, and in intervention.

In order to accomplish this purpose, a foundation of understanding the nature of humor is a logical first step. An overview of the varied and conflicting theories, the issues, controversies, and past studies will form the first part of this book.

Section II takes a look at the current utilization of humor in health settings and by the helping professionals. What purpose does humor serve? How does it fit into the usual pattern of communication? How does "medical" humor (between staff) differ from humor used with patients or clients? How has humor been used in mental health, or in education as a therapeutic tool?

If one is to make conscious use of humor, what variables would need to be considered if the attempt is to be constructive and successful? Does everyone have a "sense of humor?" How is it acquired? Is one "born" with a sense of humor or is it "developed?" Does age make a difference in appreciating humor? Do the personalities of the individuals involved make a difference? Does the culture of the patient make a difference?

Finally, although much more investigation and research needs to be conducted, some beginning guidelines for cultivating the use of humor are suggested. Elements of comedy and techniques for producing comedy are gleaned from the works of comedy writers and comedians, and developed as a guide for creating humor. There are suggestions for incorporating humor in the teaching-learning process to aid learning and to serve as a model for students, as well as for teaching the concept of humor and the utilization of humor as a tool in intervention in the helping process.

Many believe that humor is essential to human welfare and serves as a survival mechanism to cope with the "heavies of living." In the enthusiasm and urging that we not lose this great benefit, we may end up appearing to propose a "prescription" or "recipe," to humor, which may seem too mechanical. Actually, these "prescriptions" are the plant food and fertilizer to aid in the growth of humor.

The key word to remember is "cultivate." We can teach or facilitate the learning of and the knowledge about the concept of humor, but the attitude, the "sense of humor" must be enculturated. Cultivation implies the atmosphere, patience, and loving care, with the occasional application of artificial aids for revitilization and stimulation.

A companion concept which has been suggested is that of "habituation." The cultivation of humor requires consistent exposure and practice. Together with the understanding of the concept of humor, the "sense of humor" comes into bloom.

*He who laughs, lasts.* ANON

# Acknowledgments

Although my interest in humor goes way back, my first research in this area originated with a Western Council for Higher Education in Nursing project in which representatives from 24 schools of nursing met to develop mental health concepts for integrating into nursing curricula. That group collected anecdotes, shared their humor, and reviewed initial drafts of my first study. I would like to acknowledge their support. Appreciation is due to Marguerite Cobb who critiqued my work midway in the project and first encouraged me to write a book. I would also like to thank Thelma M. Schorr who provided editorial consultation on the final draft and dared us to have some original thoughts! That material became Chapter 7 of *Behavioral Concepts and Nursing Intervention* published by J. B. Lippincott in 1970.

I would also like to acknowledge the enthusiastic support and participation from 1965-1970, during that initial study, of the faculty of the School of Nursing of the University of Northern Colorado, the staff of Weld County General Hospital and the nursing students who lived through our humorous attempts.

My research in humor during my doctoral studies, which culminated in this book, was achieved through the innovative School of Educational Change and Development at the University of Northern Colorado.

I would like to extend a very special thank you to Dr. Donald G. Decker, first Dean of the school, for his initial encouragement and warm support, and to Dr. Donald M. Luketich, present Dean, who continued that support.

To my Resource Board, I will always be indebted. Their careful and provocative thought, their guidance, encouragement, and good humor supported me throughout my doctoral studies and in the writing of this book. Dr. Franklin D. Cordell supervised my progress and guided the development of the research projects. Dr. John W. Harrison steadfastly and diligently reviewed and critiqued each chapter and provided guidance and references in the area of Black Humor and comedy. Dr. Lola J. Montgomery supervised the area of personality and the sense of humor.

To my four consultants, Dr. Barbara H. Mickey, Dr. Eunice M. Blair, Dean Elaine McMinn, and Assistant Dean Elda S. Popiel, who gave of their time and expertise in special areas, I am most grateful. Dr. Mickey first suggested the narrowing of the research and guided the development of the culture research.

I would also like to thank the faculty and students at the University of Colorado School of Nursing and all the many colleagues in the community agencies who participated in the two studies. Specifically, I would like to thank Pat Meechan, Nancy Zalewski, Joanne Ruth, and Bobby Taylor who shared their studies as graduate students; Virginia Corozza, Sophronia Williams, Jessie Baus, Lydia Pourier, and Mary Drake who shared their thoughts and experiences in the development of the chapter on culture; Patsy Perry, Maureen Rausch, Margaret Ball, Carole Anderson, Gwen Stephans, and Margaret Williams whose comments and humorous examples in teaching I have used; and Signe Cooper and Mary F. Hill whose humor I have related. To all the other many, many colleagues, friends, students and patients over the years who provided me with jokes, references, and examples of humor, who participated in my studies, who reacted to my writing, laughed at my jokes, and encouraged me, I would like to express my heartfelt appreciation. I wish I could name them all, but that would be another book in itself.

Finally, but not least, I wish to acknowledge my family: husband Frank, daughters Elizabeth and Elaine, son Bill, and my mother. Without their love, support, prodding, and jokes, I would never have made it to this point of completion.

# About the Author

Vera M. Robinson, R.N., Ed.D., is Professor Emeritus, retired chair of the Department of Nursing, California State University, Fullerton. She has been a nurse educator since 1951.

A graduate of Western Pennsylvania Hospital, School of Nursing, 1944, she received her B.A. in Psychology from the University of New Mexico, 1950; her M. Litt. in Psychiatric Nursing in 1951 at the University of Pittsburgh; and her Ed.D. in Education from the University of Northern Colorado, 1975.

Dr. Robinson's pioneering research , publications and speaking in the area of humor and health has garnered her the title of the 'Fairy Godmother of Humor.' *Humor and the Health Professions* is considered a classic in the field of humor research.

# Introduction

*To everything there is a season, and a time to every purpose under heaven: a time to weep, and a time to laugh; a time to mourn, and a time to dance.*

Ecclesiastes 3:4

The past two decades have seen an increasing emphasis within the helping professions on a more humanistic approach to the individual. We recognize each person as a psychosocial being with unique motivations and behaviors. In times of illness and stress, we focus on relating to the patient as a human being, not just a biological organism. We accept him as he is and where he is, with all his problems, weaknesses, and deficiencies, as well as his strengths. We accept him as a person worthy of our respect, our caring, and our understanding. Essentially, we accept his humanness; that is, we accept not only his potential for success, but his potential for failure, his potential for tragedy, and his potential for comedy.

Within this humanistic framework of openness, caring, and warmth, humor is a natural phenomenon. As the person's self-concept develops, and he becomes more tolerant and more understanding of himself and others, he is more able to laugh at himself and at his imperfections, and to share this common bond with others.

In the helping professions, we have analyzed many human behaviors: anxiety, frustration, conflict, aggression. We have recognized the need of human beings to cry and to grieve, and have investigated the grieving process extensively. We have not however, given the same degree of attention to grief's counterpart: the need to laugh.

Yet humor and laughter are as common and pervasive as other behaviors. In fact, humor is a way of life in our society. It permeates every aspect of our existence. Observe any group in any setting —at home, at work, at play, in the street, at the office, at the factory, in the prison, the sick room, even in the funeral home, and you will hear laughter and humorous interchange. The humor may range from a smile and a simple pleasantry, to a joke-telling, slapstick session, but it is there. Humor appears in times of happiness and in times of tragedy.

Humor is one of life's great paradoxes. Humor is fun! It delights us! We love to laugh. Yet, humor is also one of the human beings most therapeutic mechanisms. It helps us to cope with life's stresses, with all the "heavies" of living. It is both pleasure and therapy.

The world we live in is full of stress. Beyond wars, earthquakes, violence and death, life is full of little daily "hassles" which are more apt to "get you" and "may be even more important in adaptation and health." (Lazarus & Folkman, 1984, p. 13) There are all those little irritations like fighting the traffic, the battle of the bulge, chores at home, bureaucracy at work, too much to do and too little time.

As health professionals and the patients who find themselves there, we also live in another world, a strange and crazy world of health care with its almost unrelenting crises, stresses and hassles. We not only face the stress of illness and its suffering — the traumas, emergencies, disabilities and death — but we must also deal with all the stress and hassles related to the environment and to the management of care. There are the daily hassles of intimate, foreboding procedures, loss of privacy, bedpans, technology, beeping monitors, overwork, understaffing, code blues and code browns.

Yet, over thousands of years, human beings have faced and survived similar stresses and hassles (Fighting dinosaurs instead of traffic?). We have survived because the human being has a built in mechanism for homeostasis, for equilibrium, for balance. One of these mechanisms we have identified is humor and its companion response — laughter.

Laughter is a biological phenomenon. As human beings we have the ability to laugh, just as we have the ability to cry. Both are the body's natural built-in response to stress, and, both provide the emotional and physical relief we need. Our ability to laugh is also related to our inherent capacity for play and to our ability to communicate. Humorous communication is the stimulus for the feeling of mirth which produces that burst of laughter. Childhood's playful laughter becomes intellectual play in adulthood.

And, whatever the physical response may be — a feeling of amusement, a smile, a giggle, a chuckle, or a big gaffaw — it is therapeutic. Humor restores our perspective, dissipates tension, frustration and fear, and produces a positive biochemical change in the body.

Yet in the past, we have given very little consideration to humor's serious functions. Although we valued the sense of humor, and listed it as an important criteria in every job description, in leadership qualities, in teaching, and as an indicator of emotional maturity, we did little to capitalize on how this great benefit could be learned and cultivated. Certainly, in the health professions, we made little planned use of humor as a communication tool for coping with stress or as a catalyst in the teaching-learning process.

Actually, in health care, we have been programmed, socialized and educated not to laugh. "Illness is a serious business—it is not a laughing matter!" Perhaps the kind of humor that occurs is another reason for its rejection. The humor if often raunchy, sexual, scatalogical, aggressive and "gallows," that is, macabre, black, gross, — often referred to as our "medical" humor. The nature of humor, however, is that it is always relevant to the situation, and we are dealing with illness, naked bodies, blood, guts, excrement, trauma and death!

Yet the humor and laughter has always been there, even though it was not sanctioned by the system. It persists! It surfaces in every area — between patients, between staff and in the interactions of health professionals with patients. Why does it occur? Because humor serves a vital purpose! It has been identified as a major coping mechanism, used by staff and patients for managing the many stresses encountered in the health care system. It has great social, psychological and physical benefits. To paraphase: Humor is not just a laughing matter. It is a serious business!

To say that humor should be taken seriously is another paradox. Humor itself is not serious. But that may be one of its greatest powers — that it is fun. This paradox may also be another reason we have avoided studying humor. It is fragile. And, because we need it desperately, we are afraid we will lose it. However, once we pass through the analytic stage and understand humor, should we not be more spontaneous, as with any other concept, and actually appreciate humor and use it therapeutically?

Martin Grotjahn contends that "he who understands the comic begins to understand humanity and the struggle for freedom and happiness." Grotjahn expresses the hope "that we may laugh even more merrily and with greater inner freedom when we understand laughter better." (Grotjahn, 1957, p. vii-ix)

This book is a beginning effort in this direction: to pull together the vast amount of literature into a body of knowledge; to make application to its use in health care; to suggest beginning guidelines for cultivating the use of humor; to incorporate it in our interactions and in our interventions with our patients and clients; and in our professional lives.

The health care field is faced today with ever increasing technological and scientific advances which threaten the very humanism of the individual — the thought of being replaced by or becoming an extension of the machine. Health professionals have been accused of caring for the machines rather than the patients.

As John Naisbitt points out in his book, *Megatrends*, for every new and complex technological advance that emerges in our society, "there must be a counterbalancing human response—that is, "high touch" and "the more high tech, the more high touch." (1982, p. 39) Humor is one of those human responses. It restores the human touch, the caring, to the highly technical, potentially dehumanizing world of health care.

# SECTION 1
## THE NATURE OF HUMOR

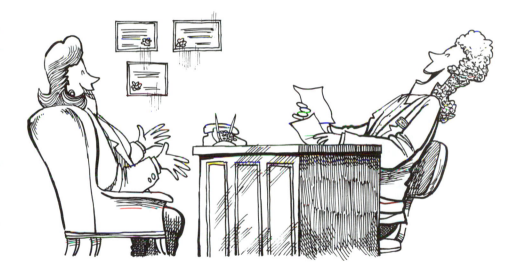

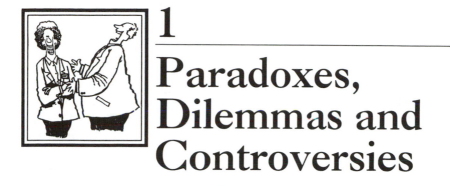

# 1
# Paradoxes, Dilemmas and Controversies

What is humor? What is the nature of humor? What is it that makes us laugh? Why does the human being need to laugh? These are the questions that have been pondered for centuries.

> Comedy . . . has been one of mankind's persistent modes of thought, of action, of self-awareness. Men have always written comedies; they have, as well, tried to explain why. No single satisfactory answer has emerged (Felheim, 1962, p. v).

The concept of humor has been considered and discussed as far back as humans could express themselves in writing — and probably long before that. Humor has been discussd by philosophers, psychologists, psychotherapists, anthropologists, sociologists, physiologists, dramatists, poets, playwrights, prose writers, satirists, comedians, educators, child development specialists, industrial management specialists ad infinitum. It seems no area of human behavior or endeavor has ignored the concept of humor and laughter.

All have attempted to define and categorize humor; to describe its nature, its causes, its effects, its purposes, and usefulness; to analyze the elements which produce it and, of course, to create it. Yet there is no consensus, and researchers and theorists continue to emphasize the difficulties of defining humor, the neglect of research and empirical evidence, and the lack of a comprehensive theory of laughter and humor (Apte, 1985 p. 13, 23; Goldstein, 1987, p. 2; Morreall, 1983 p. x).

As a matter of fact, so much has been speculated upon that each new author or theorist feels compelled to review all the past literature and thoughts before he attempts his own. Somehow, the same unique pattern occurs: the author first apologizes for the complexities involved in discussing this subject and then proceeds to present each of the past theories or writings in turn. Each theory appears to have a quality of reasonableness and validity but, as the reader is nodding his head in agreement, the author promptly tears that theory apart and proves its inadequacy. By the time the author arrives at his own theory, which he says is an attempt to bring some order out of the chaos and provide a better explanation of the nature of humor, the reader is exhausted and thoroughly confused.

The situation becomes so ludicrous that one wonders if this is not a joke on humanity by Nature, who is holding her sides in helpless laughter at man's attempt to analyze that phenomenon he has defined in terms of the ludicrous!

It has the quality of a Robert Frost:

> Forgive, Oh Lord, my little jokes on thee,
> and I'll forgive thy great big one on me(1962).

However, it soon becomes apparent that the difficulty lies in the fact that each has been attempting to find a single all-inclusive answer, when in reality, there are many answers to the nature and purpose of humor. Like many other concepts of human behavior, humor is very complex.

One of the biggest dilemmas in this area of humor is caused by the fact that there is no universally accepted language or theoretical framework. Essentially, it cuts across so many disciplines and areas of study that it belongs nowhere, yet everywhere. Each discipline ends up defining humor from its own perspective, which is never complete in itself.

Esar (1989) suggests that humor is a distinct science — a "science of humanity" — and has coined it "Humorology."

There is a dilemma in the use of terminology related to definition and to theory. There are theories which describe the nature of humor. Others relate to the purpose of humor. There are others that describe the nature of laughter. Some are proposed as theories of humor while others are presented as theories of laughter. We find that humor and laughter are used interchangeably — along with all the other words that fit into the context of humor. One cannot discuss the one without discussing the other, yet the two terms are not synonymous.

Humor is a cognitive experience, while laughter is a physical and physiologic experience. Humor is really the stimulus which produces that physical response. Humor is a form of communication; laughter is a behavior. However, to get from one to the other, there is an interim process that must occur: a perception of "funniness" and a feeling of amusement, of mirth, pleasantness, joy, surprise or absurdity. Without this emotionality of amusement or mirth, there is no laughter. Technically, the joke is still a piece of humor even if we do not find it "funny." Laughter also may occur , not in response to anything considered humorous, but in response to disease, to psychosis, or to sarcasm. We speak of the "nervous giggle‘, the sardonic laugh, playful laughter and then mirthful laughter! The core element is this feeling of mirth, an emotional process that we have not — perhaps cannot — describe theoretically, but is often recognized and alluded to in theories of humor or laughter. Freud (1903, 1928) described humor's purpose as turning "pain into pleasure;" Morreall (1983) sums up his theory of laughter as "laughter results from a pleasant psychological shift" (p.39), and Fry refers consistently in his writings to "mirth as a common and widespread emotional experience" (1977). In reporting his research on "humor physiology" (or gelotology: the science of laughter), he states:

> There are three basic elements in this system: the stimulus (humor, comedy, etc); the emotional response (mirth), and the accompanying behavior (laughter, smiling, chortling, guffawing, tittering, giggling, etc.) (1981, p. 83).

Yet, we continue to use the basic elements interchangeably or end up, as I have done in this study, using the term "humor" as an encompassing concept which includes the three-phase process plus all the other related words and behaviors! Humor is a complex cognitive, psychological and physiological phenomenon.

The nature of humor itself creates yet another dilemma in research. It poses problems in studying, analyzing and collecting data.

As we have said before, humor is a paradox in many ways. Humor requires a spontaneity, an element of surprise. There is a spontaneity-thoughtfulness balance" (Fry, 1963). If we become too thoughtful or too self-conscious about humor, we lose it. Once we stop to analyze a joke, it is no longer funny! Have you ever tried to explain a joke to someone who did not "get it?"

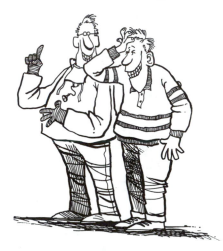

Humor can be dissected, as a frog can, but, the thing dies in the process and the innards are discouraging to any but the pure scientific mind (E. B. White).

Play also requires this same spontaneity-thoughtfulness balance, and there is a relationship between humor and play. Both are imbued with a feeling of enjoyment, fantasy, and freedom because it avoids realism. Play and humor are "not real"; it is "just fun", or it is "just a joke." Both are looked on as "trivial"; yet both function within very definite rules and a serious undertone. Humor is the only form of play usually acceptable in a predominantly serious situation.

> Behind the smoke screen of the official definition of humor as trivial, humor functions as a mode of indirect communication in the most serious of matters (Emerson, 1963, p. 10).

There is almost no situation in life — not even in dying — about which humor is not possible. Yet the responsibility associated with the seriousness is absolved in humor. One can retreat with, "I was just joking. I really didn't mean it."

Another paradox in the concept of humor is created by its subjective quality. Humor is very individual. What is funny to one person may not be funny at all to another.

Not only is this a result of the individual's own uniqueness, but humor is also situational. Humor flows out of the interaction within a particular situation or setting. To appreciate that humor requires a knowledge of the setting, the situation, the event, or the society or culture. There may be a need for background information. The persons involved may react with hilarity, but an outsider may wonder, "What was so funny?"

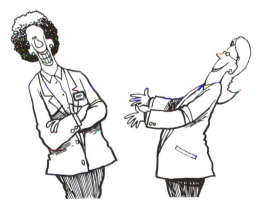

In a lecture on brain tumors, the instructor was discussing the methods for pinpointing the location of the tumor and the importance of doing so prior to surgery. She said "You can grub around in an abdomen, but you can't grub around in a brain!" The students roared with laughter. But, to the lay person, who did not understand the anatomy and physiology involved and the ludicrousness of "grubbing" in the brain, this comment might even be repugnant, let alone unfunny.

These paradoxes create difficulties in attempts to observe and study humor, or collect data in natural as well as laboratory settings. Empirical studies to validate theoretical constructs about humor are often questioned because there are not enough data from natural setting to provide a norm against which studies can be judged.

In direct observation of any communication, we know that the presence of another person affects that interaction. When humor is known to be the topic of observation, one of two reactions occur. Either the person or group becomes so self-conscious that the humor disappears, or quite the opposite occurs (which is another paradox), the quantity of humor increases. People try harder to be funny. Humor is contagious. One joking comment leads to another.

Joan Emerson (1963), in her doctoral study investigating the social functions of humor in a hospital setting, spent eight months collecting data. She said:

> To observe relatively unself-conscious interaction it was necessary to stay in one setting long enough to accustom the subjects to the presence of the observer.

Emerson sat in on the course for nurse's aides so that she could participate in the ongoing activity while observing the interactions of the staff with the patients. She had to be available and as unobtrusive a part of the normal routine as possible in order to be there when the humor occurred. And yet, her observer's role was often regarded as a joking matter and her following the subjects around provoked humor.

The other approach to collecting data in natural settings is to ask the individuals within the settings to record their own humorous interactions. This poses another problem. Since humor is more often spontaneous and situational, the individual gets "caught up" in the exchange and forgets to record. Later, when one tries to recall the incident, it is often difficult to remember the details, unless it was exceptionally funny. The banter or jocular talk gets lost. Or, this kind of humorous interaction was such an integral part of the communication pattern that the participant does not relate to the fact of humor, or consider it a humorous incident. Often, the person will say, "They laughed, but I don't know what I did that was so funny!"

Thus the collected results may be meager, and because the researcher was not in the situation, reading the observations, he may have difficulty seeing "what was funny."

Because collecting original data in natural settings becomes a long and difficult process, others have attempted to control situations by experimental studies in the laboratory. This obviously creates problems in terms of the spontaneity, and raises the question of salience; that is, whatever happens to be the topic presented is the one that arouses the humor. When you put laughter in a laboratory, is the laughter forced because the subjects are expected to laugh? Is the humor to which they are exposed funny to the researcher, but not really funny to the subjects?

Laboratory studies measure response to artificial humor rather than the spontaneous, naturally created humor as it occurs in a natural setting. Generalizing from observations in the natural settings has its bias as well, but the participants negative responses are "natural" and negative responses and failed humor can also be observed. Reliable methodological tools for studying spontaneous humor and tools for measuring long term effects are also an issue. The physiologic effects of laughter may be easier to measure than humor — which is cognitive. The controversy over qualitative and quantitative research continues in this area of humor. Perhaps one of the major dilemmas in this study of humor (like other concepts such as love, joy, hope) is that they are complex emotions with so many related behaviors that they do not lend themselves to rigid experimental scientific methodology. Once you do, you lose that essence, that feeling that is the quintessence of the phenomenon itself.

> "What are we to make of all the paradoxes in humor theory . . . ? The answer is, I believe, that we are just beginning to accept how important, how complex and difficult, and how varied the study of humor can be and the answers are still out there" (Mintz, 1988, p. ix-x).

Despite all the dilemmas, the controversies and issues in research, the studies do go on (McGhee & Goldstein 1983). Humor is a phenomenon which continues to intrigue mankind.

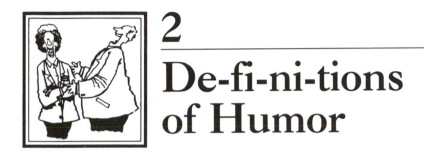

# 2
# De-fi-ni-tions
# of Humor

Finding a universal definition for humor is as difficult as finding a universal language or theory. Most authors simply avoid the issue by not defining it. Humor scholars have not been able to agree on a central definition; humor is an elusive concept for which a precise definition may not be possible and most efforts have not been successful. Yet each of us must provide the parameters of that concept we are describing.

Webster's dictionary defines humor as "that quality which appeals to a sense of the ludicrous or absurdly incongruous" and lists the archaic definition of humor (umor) as "moisture, vapor."

In old medieval physiology, humor referred to the four principal fluids of the body: blood, phlegm, cholor (yellow bile), and melancholy (black bile). The predominance of any of these fluids determined man's health or temperment or mood. A just balance made a good compound called "good humor," and a preponderance of any one made a bad compound called "ill humor." We still speak of a person's "good humor."

Others in the past have defined humor from their own particular perspectives. Crothers called humor the "frank enjoyment of the imperfect." Stephen Leacock defined it as the "kindly contemplation of the incongruities of life and the artistic contemplation thereof."

Evan Esar, whose *Comic Dictionary* is in its 4th Edition, (1983), defines humor, among others, as "fun that's funny" and, "the hole that lets the sawdust out of the stuffed shirt." He also defines laughter as "the sensation of feeling good all over and showing it principally in one place."

Most definitions of humor are described in relation to laughter, with laughter as the indicator that humor has occurred. As we have said before, the two words are often used to describe each other and interchangeably. It is further complicated by the emotional response of amusement or mirth or perception of funny, which is an inherent part of the process.

To add to the complexity, there are many other behavioral responses which are also considered indications of amusement: smiling, a twinkling of the eyes, change in facial expression, or a giggle, chortle, guffaw or groan. And, there are a myriad of related terms to describe humor which many have attempted to distinguish, such as wit, satire, punning, clowning, teasing, joking, comedy, pantomime, banter, sarcasm, cartoons, etc.

So, like all the others, not to be snared in the trap of attempting all these distinctions, a more generic definition will provide for the breadth and varieties of humor which can occur in the natural setting, and can incorporate the emotional component in identifying the functions of humor, its purpose. Since humor is being viewed as a medium of communication in health settings, it will be more useful to define humor as any communication which is perceived by any of the interacting parties as humorous and leads to laughing, smiling and a feeling of amusement. Humor will also be used in this book as a broad concept incorporating the three part process of humor as a cognitive communication leading to an emotional response of amusement, pleasure and mirth, which results in a behavioral physical response of laughter and its counterparts.

Humor as a form of communication has also been further defined. Most of the humor within health settings is spontaneous or situational in nature rather than the formal joke-telling or practical joke variety. Formal humor may be cartoons, literary works, planned inclusions of jokes, or funny stories in speeches, lectures or other structured situations. Spontaneous humor, on the other hand, arises out of ordinary situations and is usually a witty remark or ludicrous action inspired by the circumstances at hand. Its success depends on the right moment and right circle of participants (Emerson, 1963, p. 11-12).

Spontaneous humor has been further defined as "jocular remarks" which consist of two forms: pleasantries and witticisms. A pleasantry is a mild form of humor to which no laughter may be attached. It may be simply a humorous turn of phrase, an attempt to be pleasant by being mildly amusing. A witticism, on the other hand, makes a greater attempt to entertain. It is more clever and original. "Pleasantries are little bubbles coming to the surface of the water and disappearing, a witticism makes a loud splash" (Emerson, p. 137).

William Fry (1963) gives a similar division. He defines spontaneous humor as situation jokes, which have their origin in the ongoing interpersonal process. Canned jokes are those presented with little obvious relationship to the ongoing human interaction. Practical jokes are a combination of both, in that they are consciously contrived but depend on the unfolding of an interpersonal interaction for the humor to occur.

Avner Ziv (1983, 1989) has proposed categorizing humor as intentional or voluntary, as opposed to unintentional or involuntary. Intentional humor is that humor created by people in order to be enjoyed. Unintentional humor is when the person had no intention of making others laugh, but it happens. It can be non-verbal, like slipping on a banana peel or other ludicrous behavior, or verbal, like a slip of the tongue, or a child's naive remark or a malapropism (1983, 1989).

All of these kinds of humor occur in health care and will be described and discussed in the sections "Humor in Health and Illness" and "Cultivating the Use of Humor."

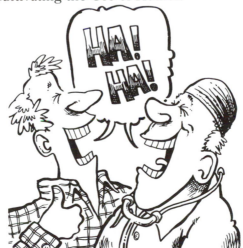

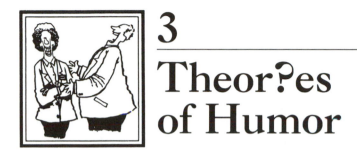

# 3
# Theor?es
# of Humor

Despite the lack of consensus as to theory and despite the formidable task of attempting to review all the literature, I am as undaunted, and as apologetic, as all the previous authors. In the absence of a single framework to which to relate, not having this overall background knowledge would seem to be like embarking on a trip without a map.

However, this chapter only attempts an overview of the theories in the development of the major thesis of this book. Most theories, research and studies will be discussed in other chapters in relation to specific areas. For those who wish even greater depth, the original works and other reviews are available. (Flugel, 1954; Keith-Speigel, 1971; Morreall, 1983, 1987; Haig, 1988) (If however, you are a free spirit who prefers to travel unburdened by maps, you are at liberty to move on!)

Many of the writings about humor have not offered pure theories as such. Many of them have included analyses of specific characteristics of humor. Many have been speculations as to the nature of humor or the functions of humor. Many are classics in the field which have cogent insights to add to the basic understanding of humor and so are included in any discussion of theory.

This multifaceted review poses a problem in how to categorize these theories. Consequently, three approaches have been used. One has been to do a chronological, historical accounting by years or centuries. A second method is to review by discipline: philosophy, psychology, sociology, etc. The third approach is to present by functional or issue categories. I shall summarize from each of the last two approaches.

# PERSPECTIVES FROM THE HUMANITIES

The humanities and the literature of the world, with its comedy writers and critics from the ancient Greeks to the present, have been concerned with the nature of comedy and laughter. Comedy reveals man's imperfections, leaves him more tolerant, and gives him the courage to face life. This is the theme of most comedy writers and comedians. Comedy is not just a happy as opposed to an unhappy ending, but a way of surveying life. All tragedy is idealistic and says "the pity of it," while comedy tends to be skeptical and says, "the absurdity of it" (Kronenberger, 1952).

> In mortal affairs it is tragedy, like forgiveness, that seems divine, and comedy, like error, that is human (p. 194).

Steve Allen (1981) contends that "without laughter life on our planet would be intolerable" (p. 201). Laughter, he says, is so important to us that "humanity highly rewards . . . . those who make a living by inducing laughter in others." Elements of comedy and styles of humor — what makes people laugh and how to create it — has been the focus of others, and studies of comedy writers and of comedians have revealed the essence of this creativity. (Fry & Allen, 1975; Allen, 1981, 1982, 1987; Fisher & Fisher, 1983; Helitzer, 1984; Orben, 1963, 1987).

# PHILOSOPHICAL PERSPECTIVES

Early philosophers were primarily concerned with the nature of humor in relation to the nature of man, and the issue of good and evil. Does humor represent the best in man or the worst? Plato and Aristotle felt that humor was the enjoyment of the misfortunes of others and comedy was an imitation of men at their worst. Other philosophers viewed laughter as a weapon against evil and a valuable asset in correcting the minor follies of society (Hazlitt, Dryden).

Morreall (1983, 1987) felt that the negative evaluation of humor by the early Greek philosophers hampered the study and development of humor theory. The major theories of the past are all just part of one general theory and he proposes a formula for a comprehensive theory of laughter: laughter results from a pleasant psychological shift.

There are two ingredients in Morreall's theory. One, that there is a change of a psychological state, which can be cognitive/perceptual or affective/emotional, and change must be sudden (a shift), and, two, that it must be pleasant. His is a theory of laughter, he says, because it is the physical activity which is the end result and that laughter is the natural expression of amusement.

## PSYCHOANALYTIC PERSPECTIVES

The psychoanalytic theory of humor originated by Sigmund Freud has been one of the major frameworks for the study of humor. Freud became interested in jokes when he became aware of the similarites between the technique of jokes and dreams. His analysis resulted in his book, *Jokes and their relation to the unconscious* (1905). There are two types of jokes: the harmless joke, and the joke with a purpose or "tendentious" wit. Civilization has produced repression of many basic impulses, Freud says, and joking becomes a socially acceptable way of satisfying those needs. He described four major types of purposeful jokes: the sexual joke, the aggressive, hostile joke, the blasphemous joke, and the skeptical joke. The process is an unconscious one and there is a saving of psychic energy.

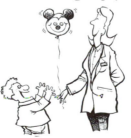

Freud differentiates between wit, the comic effect, and humor. However, all have the same motif, that of economy. The pleasure of wit originates from the economy of inhibition, the comic from an economy of thought, and humor from an economy of feelings. This effect strives to reproduce the state of childhood when our expenditure of psychic energy was slight and we did not need all these jokes, humor and comic effects to "make us feel happy in our life."

Freud also developed a theory of laughing at tragedy and death, called "gallows humor", which has been the basis for much study since and will be discussed later in relation to medical humor.

In a short article published in 1928, Freud developed further his concept of humor. Humor has something liberating about it, is not resigned. The ego refuses to be distressed by reality, to let itself suffer. It is a triumph of narcissism through the indulgence of the superego, yet does not overstep the bounds of mental health. Not everyone, Freud says, is capable of this rare and precious gift, however.

Many of the studies and other theories since then have been built on the basis of Freud's theory — that humor has a major psychological purpose as a relief mechanism.

# PSYCHOLOGICAL PERSPECTIVES

Psychologists have dealt primarily with the individual in defining humor, i.e., why one individual laughs and not another. They have also focused on laboratory-controlled experiments rather than arm-chair theorizing or studies in natural settings. They have looked at such personality traits as aggression, sex, creativity, and intelligence, among others, in understanding humor, as well as to the presence or development of a "sense of humor." Much of this work has used Freud's theory as a base.

More recently, psychologists have become concerned with the lack of any systematic empirical and theoretical attack on humor and have voiced the belief that, although psychoanalytic theory has made a significant contribution, it is limited in its capacity to stimulate further advancement (Goldstein & McGhee, 1972). The new approach is built around arousal and cognitive factors (Berlyne, 1972; Suls, 1972, 1983). Humor is not simply determined by the present stimulus situation but depends on recollections of the past and anticipations of the future. It is a collative process which is important in generating or arousing the pleasure of humor. The processing is cognitively based; it also involves information-processing and problem-solving ability. We must perceive the incongruity and resolve it before we "get the joke."

Harvey Mindess (1971) proposes another theory which, he says, encompasses all others. He calls it the liberation theory. He sees humor and laughter as the agent of psychological liberation. It frees us from the constraints and restrictive forces of daily living and in doing so, makes us joyful. He urges us to cultivate our sense of humor and provides us with some thoughts on how to achieve this.

Lefcourt and Martin (1986) proposed that humor was a modifier of stress; that humor and laughter play a major role in the maintenance of both psychological and physiological health and well being in the face of life's stresses. Because empirical investigation was needed to support that premise, they developed an assessment tool for measuring the individual's sense of humor: the Situational Humor Response Questionnaire, and the Coping Humor Scale to assess the degree to which individuals make use of humor in coping with stress.

# ANTHROPOLOGICAL PERSPECTIVES

The main contributions of the anthroplogists have been to describe the humor components within cultures or ethnic groups as a part of their investigations. Radcliffe-Brown's early (1940) identification of the joking relationships between kin members greatly influenced other research. He defined the joking relationship as a:

> . . . . relation between two persons in which one is by custom permitted, and, in some instances required, to tease or make fun of the other, who in turn is required to take no offense (p. 90).

It is "permitted disrespect," a combination of friendliness and antagonism. This kind of social relationship is widespread in other societies and the concept provides a base for comparative studies of social structures.

Apte (1985) provides the first cross-cultural study of humor from an anthropological perspective. Humor, he says, is the result of cultural perceptions, both individual and collective. Humor is a cognitive experience which must have a cultural niche and cannot occur in a vacuum.

Dundes (1987) has studied joking and joking cycles as a folklorist. He believes that no piece of folklore continues to be transmitted unless it has meaning, yet the joke's meaning must not be crystal clear. If people knew what they were communicating, the "jokes would cease to be effective as socially sanctioned outlets for expressing taboo ideas and subjects" (p.vii). In any society where there is anxiety, there will be jokes to express it; when there is political repression, there will be political jokes.

Humor is universal, but the culture, society or ethnic group in which it occurs will make a difference in the style, the contents of humor and the situations in which humor is used and considered appropriate (Ziv, 1988).

# SOCIOLOGICAL PERSPECTIVES

Although the sociologists have been the last group to get involved in the concept of humor, their contributions have been increasing. Perhaps, the first sociological theory was offered in 1900 by Henri Bergson who described the nature of humor as "the mechanical encrusted on the living." A person is laughable when he behaves in a rigid, automatic way. Humor functions as a social corrective on this unadaptive behavior. The comic, Bergson says, does not exist outside the pale of the human. Laughter is always within a group and must remain in touch with other intelligent beings. Laughter functions to socialize the individual into a group and groups into society.

Others credit Obrdlik's (1942) study on the phenomenon of gallows humor in Nazi-occupied Czechoslovakia as the first to deal with humor in a sociological framework. The humor served a social function in bolstering morale of the oppressed group while disintegrating the forces against whom the humor was directed. The humor made the fear and tragedy seem temporary.

Humor is a social relationship and occurs in a social environment, and the role of humor in this context has been studied by many (Fine, 1983). Humor promotes group cohesion, and initiates relationships. Studies have emphasized the control function of humor as a means of expressing approval or disapproval of social action, and to relieve tension in social conflict (Stephenson, 1951).

The role of the fool and the clown in society has been described as a lowly one, yet valued. The fool serves as a scapegoat and as a means of enforcing group norms of propriety. Studies of the social functions of humor in race relations and in ethnic and other minority groups describe the function of humor as solidifying the in-group, to attain gratification at the expense of another group, as a way to reduce the prejudice, create a new image, and as an agent for social change (Boskin, 1979). The social functions and joking relationships in organizations which serve to minimize the stress and release the antagonism, including those within the health care setting, have also been studied. These will be discussed in that section.

# SUPERIORITY THEORIES

The superiority theory has been described as one of the classic, traditional theories of humor. Some have felt that this element is an ingredient in all humor.

The basis of the superiority theory lies in the assertion of our own superiority by laughing at the inferiority, stupidity, or misfortunes of others. Plato and Aristotle reflected this pleasure in the pain of others. Thomas Hobbs in 1893 defined laughter as a "sudden glory arising from some sudden conception of some eminency in ourselves by comparison with the infirmity of others." Bergson's theory of "the mechanical encrusted on the living" views humor as laughing at the stereotyped, unsocial behavior of others. Ridicule and laughter at the foolish actions of others are reflected in the clown, Charlie Chaplin, Laurel and Hardy, the Keystone Kops, the pie-in-the-face, slipping-on-the-banana peel type of comedy. There is the sense of aggression, "a roar of triumph . . . " (Rapp, 1951). Others believe that this laughter is not always cruel and scornful, but may be a laughter of warmth and empathy as well. Essentially, we are laughing at ourselves, at our own imperfections. For that moment we feel superior. It did not happen to us, but it could! Meeker (1974) asserts that comedy demonstrates "that man is durable, even though he may be weak, stupid, and undignified" (p.24).

This theory of superiority has also been called the disparagement theory, the ability to laugh at ourselves, at our own inferiorities. Others have described this theory as being on a continuum: from laughing at no one (nonsense, puns), to laughing at someone, specific people or groups, (moron jokes, Pollack jokes), to laughing with others in general at man's foibles, and to laughing at one's self, the most therapeutic of all. All aspects of the continuum are not merely ridicule or acts of aggression but gives a sense of mastery over the situation. This may be the key ingredient in the coping, survival function of humor and laughter.

# INCONGRUITY THEORIES

The incongruity theory has also been considered a classic, traditional theory. Surprise, ambivalence, conflict and incongruity have been words to describe this necessary element or component of the humorous experience. There must be a sudden "shock" or unexpectedness, a "surprise," an incongruity, ambivalence, or conflict of ideas or emotions which produces the absurdity resulting in a burst of laughter.

Kant in 1790 observed that laughter is "an affectation arising from the sudden transformation of a strained expectation into nothing." For Schopenhauer, laughter arises from the sudden perception of an incongruity between an object and a concept. Spencer saw laughter occurring when "the conscious is unawares transferred from great things to small — a descending incongruity." An ascending incongruity gives rise to wonder, not laughter. Bergson stated that a situation is comic when it belongs simultaneously to two altogether independent series of events and is capable of being interpreted in two entirely different meanings at the same time. Koestler (1964) attributed humor to "biosociation" — perceiving a situation or event in two habitually incompatible associated contexts. Monroe (1951) described the experience of ambivalent emotions. We laugh whenever, on contemplating an object or situation, we find opposite emotions struggling within us for mastery.

Although described as a configurational theory, these are similar to the surprise and incongruity theories. The difference is the sudden "insight" or "falling into place" that creates the laughter rather than the unexpected "disjointedness" that is the amusement of incongruity.

This concept is based on Gestalt psychology which involves perception of the whole. We begin ordering perceptions in a reasoning fashion when they are presented, but it is the unexpected configuration which results that is the surprise and whch appears ludicrous. The appreciation of a joke is related to shifts in figure-ground perception. When reversal occurs, we "get the point" of the joke.

Many other authors have identified this concept of surprise or incongruity as the necessary ingredient in the creation of humor.

# PLAY THEORIES

The element of play has also been considered a necessary component of humor. Many writers have described humor as an aspect of play, made comparisons between play and humor, or incorporated the aspect of play as a developmental factor in acquiring a sense of humor. The "playful" nature of humor and laughter is common to most theories about the nature of humor.

Sully (1902) stated that the enjoyment of the laughable comes from arousal of the play mood, a refusal to take the situation seriously, which is the characteristic feature of play. Eastman (1936) defined humor as play, stating that humor has no value except the values possessed by play. No definition or explanation of humor will hold up, he says, which is not based on a distinction between playful and serious. There must be this element of play, of being "in fun," for humor to occur.

William Fry (1963) did an extensive study of the relation of humor to play, and laughing and smiling to both. Both involve an interpersonal interaction communication, both are sensitive to the spontaneity-thoughtfulness balance, and both involve manipulation in the levels of abstraction. Fry describes the development of play and humor from birth to adulthood. He describes both as having a framework of unreality or fun, i.e., a play-frame and a joke frame. He also compares play and humor to fighting and aggression — the wrestling around and playful slaps are related to the "punch" line of the joke.

Berlyne, in his discussion of laughter, humor and play, states that laughter and play are so widespread in human societies that their absence may be judged abnormal (1969). As a matter of fact, societies expend a greater part of their time and energy in playful and humorous pursuits.

The relationship of play in the development of humor is described by McGhee (1979). The sense of humor develops in context with the social, emotional, intellectual and physical development of the child. This origin of the "sense of humor" and the research on children's humor will be discussed more fully in the section on children and humor.

# RELIEF OR RELEASE THEORIES

The theories of humor have been variously grouped as those which describe the nature of humor: the superiority theories, the incongruity theories and the play theories, and those which describe the purpose or functions of humor, called the relief or release theories. These theories have as their base the concept that humor is a relief from tension, anxiety, frustration or the release from the harsh realities of life.

Most of the theories or perspectives from the disciplines, the psychological, sociological, and philosophical as well as the biological would seem to fall in this category. The relief can be cognitive, an escape from reality, from reason. Or, it can be emotional relief from anxiety, fear, anger, embarrassment or social conflict. Or it can be a physical release of "nervous energy." Many studies have incorporated this idea of relief as one of the many functions of humor.

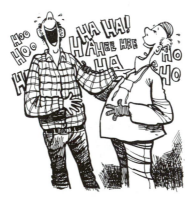

# BIOLOGICAL AND INSTINCT THEORIES

Many theorists have viewed laughter as a physiological mechanism which is "good for the body." McDougall believed that laughter was basically an "instinct" invented by nature as an antidote to our tendency to sympathize with the distress of others (1903). Laughter produces a sense of well-being and a euphoria which has a biologic "survival" value. Secondarily, he says, laughter serves a social function. The sense of humor makes us capable of laughing at our own minor misfortunes. There is also a larger humor, which finds laughter in those defects common to all men.

Koestler (1964) also describes laughter as a physiological reaction similar to tears, which seem to have no biological function yet produce such obvious relief that they can hardly be called "luxury reflexes." Koestler links laughter with comedy and describes comedy as an act of creativity.

James Walsh (1928), a physician, described laughter as "massaging" of all the organs within the body and as a potent factor in good health.

Others have described laughter as an evolutionary process beginning with the "baring of teeth" and snarling to forestall attack and developing into the smile and laugh which communicates that one can relax in safety (Hayworth, 1928). Laughter and humor have become a substitute for actual assault.

Darwin and others have described smiling and laughter, and speculated on its good to the body, but actual research on the physiological and biochemical results of laughter began when the scientific tools to measure the response became available in recent years. This research will be discussed in the chapter, "The Physiology of Laughter."

# SUMMARY

It should be apparent after this brief review why this concept of humor is so controversial. For so common a phenomenon it is extremely complex! Most theories have yet to be empirically tested and none is complete in itself. It is obvious that they overlap. Essentially, they collectively explain this concept of humor. In looking at theories, the only solution is to remain open and eclectic in trying to understand this very vital human behavior.

All the theories and perspectives from the disciplines will be integrated and applied in this study describing the use, purpose and functions of humor in health and health care.

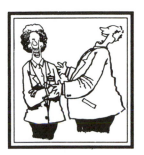

# 4

# The Physiology of Laughter and Its Therapeutic Effects

*A merry heart doeth good like a medicine: but a broken spirit drieth the bones.*

Proverbs 17:22

The physical, biological phenomenon of laughter has been described and speculated upon for centuries. Laughter has long been affirmed as necessary for biological survival and that it has health-giving properties. It is also recognized that the absence of laughter and humor and play in the human being impaired physical and psychological health (Berlyne, 1969). But it has only been in the past several decades that there has been the scientific research and the tools to begin to measure the physiological and biochemical effects of laughter on the human body.

In medieval physiology, humor was described as the four principal fluids of the body: blood, phlegm, color, and melancholy.

A balance made for "good humor." "Humor therapy" and "court jesters" were used in ancient Greece and the Middle Ages. Henri de Mondeville, a medieval professor of surgery, was a proponent of mirth as an aid to recovery, and advocated that negative emotions must not be allowed to interfere. "Let the surgeon take care to regulate the whole regime of the patient's life for joy and happiness. . . . . forbid anger, hatred and sadness in the patient, and remind him that the body grows fat from joy, and thin from sadness" (cited in Moody, 1978, p. 28-29).

In an analysis of laughter, French physician Laurent Joubert (1579) thought the contrary emotions of joy and sadness stirred the heart in alternating dilatations. This "to and fro" movement is transferred to the diaphragm, leading to the rapid breathing we call "hearty laughter." The consequences of laughter are beneficial, he says, and can be seen in the face and eyes (cited in Goldstein, 1987, p. 205-6).

Other early scholars referred to the healthful benefits of laughter and attempted to describe the physiological effects. Kant (1790) wrote, ". . . . we feel the effect of this slackening body by the oscillation of the organs, which promotes the restoration of equilibrium and has a favorable effect on health." Spencer (1860) described laughter as the discharge of excess nervous excitement. Darwin (1872/1965) stated that with laughter derived from the excitement of pleasure, "circulation becomes more rapid; the eyes are bright and the colour of the face rises. The brain being stimulated by the increased flow of blood, reacts on the mental powers" (p. 32). McDougall (1903/1963) defined laughter as an instinct that has "survival value," it "seems to quicken the respiratory and circulatory processes and . . . . to produce a general sense of well-being or euphoria (p. 338). Sully (1902/1963) suggested that laughter was good exercise and promoted good digestion.

In a classic book (1928), James Walsh, a physician, gives reasons why the "cultivation of a habit of laughter is a potent factor for health." He describes the relationship of laughter to all the body organs and systems. The principal physical agent, he says, is the diaphragm and since all the other organs are just above or below, they are "massaged" in such a way as to modify their circulation of blood. He describes the effects upon the lungs, the increase in oxidation of the blood that accomplishes "the same thorough going stimulation of inspiration as exercise with sport" (p. 37).

Koestler (1964) described laughter as a reflex. Humor is "the only domain of creativity where a stimulus on a high level of complexity produces a massive and sharply defined response on the level of physiologic reflexes" (p. 31).

Modern research began investigating the concept of arousal, humor appreciation, and the reduction of tension through laughter by measuring heart rate, muscle tension and galvanic skin responses. Averill (1969) (as cited in Godkewitsch, 1976) found increased heart rate associated with mirth and concluded that the humor experience results in arousal of the sympathetic nervous system. Schachter and Wheeler (1962) found that an increase in arousal was a necessary condition in the appreciation of humor. Subjects injected with epinephrine were more amused than control subjects injected with saline or a third group injected with chlorpromazine. Goldstein (1970), recording skeletal muscle response (reaction time), found that latencies of overt humor responses were shorter for more humorous cartoons. Langevin and Day (1972) found that galvanic skin response amplitude was positively correlated with humor appreciation. Godkewitsch (1976) concluded that arousal, as indexed by heart rate and skin conductance, increases with the intensity of the humor response.

Others began investigating the overall physiological response to laughter. What does happen in the body when we laugh? William Fry, whose research of the physiological effects of laughter has been the most comprehensive, concluded that "mirth and its mirthful behavior have impact on most of the major physiologic systems of the body" and that further study should demonstrate that mirth affects all physiological systems (Fry, 1986, p. 84). Laughter, he says, is an "aerobic experience," an internal stationary jogging!

Fry (1969, 1971, 1977 a,b, 1979) studied the effects of mirthful laughter on heart rate, oxygen saturation levels of peripheral blood and respiratory phenomena. The physiologic impact of humor is as complex as the psychological. He found that both the arousal and cathartic effects of humor are paralleled in the physiological. Laughter, in contrast to other emotions, involves extensive physical activity and the results are comparable to that of physical exercise. It increases respiratory activity and oxygen exchange, increases muscular activity and heart rate, and stimulates the cardiovascular system, the sympathetic nervous system, and the production of catecholamines.

The arousal state is followed by a relaxation state in which respiration, heart rate, and muscle tension return to below normal levels. The oxygen saturation level of peripheral blood is not affected during this relaxation state; blood pressure is reduced, and a state similar to the impact of hearty exercise exists.

Another circulatory system study (Fry & Savin, 1982) investigated further the effects of humor on arterial blood pressure using direct arterial cannulization. There were increases in systolic and diastolic blood pressure directly related to the intensity and length of the laughter. Blood pressure levels decreased immediately after the laughter decreasing to below the pre-laughter base.

Bushnell and Scheff (1979) claimed support for the catharsis theory of laughter in the demonstration of physiologic relaxation and reduction of muscle tension during hearty laughter. Svebak (1975, 1977) also investigated the respiratory phenomenon in laughter. He found that variability in the tonus of abdominal muscles of women during the inspiratory-expiratory cycle of "belly laughs" facilitated more frequent and enduring laughter responses.

In later research (Svebak, 1982) investigated the effects of humor on the brain in terms of hemispheric dominance through electro-physiological studies of brain activity. The EEG data revealed greater coordination of function between right and left hemispheres. His findings indicated that laughter stimulated both hemispheres at the same time, coordinating all the senses and producing a unique level of consciousness and a high level mode of brain processing. The brain is essentially at its fullest capacity with the right and left brain functioning simultaneously.

Gardner (1981), in studying brain-damaged patients for linguistic abilities, found that only when both hemispheres of the brain were working together can the punch line of a joke be appreciated. The left hemisphere has been considered the dominant agent in linguistic functioning, but right-hemisphere damaged patients not only crack jokes at inappropriate times, but have difficulty getting the sense of jokes as told by others.

William Frey, II, at the University of Minnesota (1985) investigated the chemical properties of tears (tears of laughter as well as grief), and found that emotional tearing is a unique exocrine response to stress similar to other excretory functions of the body. Emotional tears carry the same toxins found in cells under stress.

In a series of scientifically controlled experiments (direct venous blood sampling during exposure to humor) at Loma Linda University, Lee Berk, et al (1989) investigated the effect of laughter on the neuroendocrine, stress hormones and the immune parameters. There is a complex autonomic response with each catacholamine, suggesting that laughter may be an antagonist to the classical stress response. This study arose out of research conducted on exercise and its effects on the immune system. The laughter response simulates moderate exercise which is a eustress (good stress) rather than a distress.

Earlier research by McClelland (cited in Long, 1987) and Dillon & Baker (1985-1986) found that humor and laughter significantly increased levels of salivary immunoglobulin A, a vital immune system protein, which is the body's first line of defense against respiratory illnesses.

Other major psycho-neuroimmunological research is being conducted, on not only the effect of laughter, but on the effect of all the positive emotions on the immune system and its interactions with the brain and the endocrine system. The new research in the whole area of psycho-neuro-bio-endocrine-immunology has indicated that the brain and the immune system are a closed circuit, and that the mind and body do "talk to each other."

What are the implications of the physiological research? That laughter has a positive effect on the body and a positive effect on health. The implications of the value of laughter in prevention of disease are many, says Fry. Heart disease, cerebral vascular accidents, cancer, depression and other stress related illnesses could all be reduced (1979).

Laughter has many benefits as an adjunct to therapy in cardiac rehabilitation, in chronic diseases like arthritis and emphysema, and in the aging process (Fry, 1986. It can stimulate the circulatory system, including heart muscle, and "stir the circulation of immune elements." Since laughter is primarily an expiratory experience, it can clear the lungs of mucous and bathe the body in oxygen. It can stimulate muscles and relax muscle tension, since all the muscles of the body are involved in a good belly laugh — face, neck, chest, abdomen, arms and legs. This relaxation of muscle tension can reduce pain! The production of the catecholamines not only stimulates the production of the endorphins in the brain, the body's natural opiate, but also increases adrenaline in the brain. This stimulates alertness and memory and enhances learning and creativity. For a thorough review of the research on the physiology of laughter, and its therapeutic effects, see Fry (1986) and Goldstein (1987).

# CAN LAUGHTER HEAL?

## The Mind-Body Connection

The only documented account of healing through the use of laughter is that of Norman Cousins' (1979) widely publicized recovery from a crippling, incurable collagen disease, ankylosing spondylitis. The event occurred in 1964, but was not reported until 1976 in the *New England Journal of Medicine*.

Cousins, a former editor of *Saturday Review*, became ill following a stressful and exhausting trip abroad, and was hospitalized with fever, malaise, and increasing pain and paralysis. Reasoning that he was in a state of adrenal exhaustion, with a less than functioning immunologic system, and being familiar with Hans Seyle's theory of stress, he planned a program with his physician to replenish this system.

> If negative emotions produce negative chemical changes in the body, wouldn't the positive emotions produce positive chemical changes? Is it possible that love, hope, faith, laughter, confidence, and the will to live have therapeutic value (p. 34-35)?

Along with the elimination of all medications and massive doses of vitamin C, he programmed sessions for laughter since he "already had hope, love, faith, and the will to live."

Candid Camera and old Marx Brothers films and humor books were part of the package.

> It worked. I made the joyous discovery that ten minutes of genuine belly laughter had an anesthetic effect and would give me at least two hours of pain-free sleep (p. 39).

Following each episode, the sedimentation rate was measured. Each time, there was a drop of five to nine points. It was cumulative and there was a return to normal levels, indicating a resolution of the inflammatory process. From there, he gradually regained movement and health to complete recovery. He concluded that "there is a physiologic basis for the ancient theory that laughter is good medicine . . . . I have learned never to underestimate the capacity of the human mind and body to regenerate . . . . " (p. 48).

There have been many other anecdotal accounts of "healing" recalled by individuals, professionals, clowns, and chaplains, and reported by physicians, including Moody (1978), Simonton (1978), and Siegal (1986). These include areas of psychiatry and in life-threatening diseases like cancer and heart disease.

Norman Cousins (1983) recounts his second recovery from a massive heart attack in 1980, avoiding major by pass surgery again through his positive attitude. The key to healing, he says, is the reduction of panic, helplessness and anxiety. The mind and body are so closely related. Laughter and other positive emotions he says, are not a substitute for traditional medicine, but an adjunct to mobilizing the body's own resources and "freeing the body of the constricting effects of the negative (p. 154).

He emphasized again that laughter must be associated with love, warmth, hope, faith, the will to live, and creativity and playfulness.

Siegal, in his holistic approach to cancer patients, says "learning to love conquers the fear of death and can liberate incredible healing energy" (1986, p. 223).

Research on the long-term consequences of humor is still needed. We do know that the positive attitude seems to have prolonged the lives of those with serious illnesses, but we do not know if humor is a factor in longevity. What we have ascertained is that humor and laughter can certainly increase the quality of our lives!

# SUMMARY

The physiologic and biochemical research on humor that has occurred is an exciting breakthrough in documenting the "healthful" properties of laughter.

The important issue here is that humor is a complex cognitive, emotional, psychological and physiological phenomenon. It takes the humor to stimulate the mirthful emotion which produces the physical response of laughter and triggers the biochemical changes within the body. The study, then, of humor and how to cultivate it for emotional and physical healing will be the focus of this book.

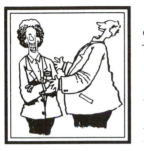

# 5
# Styles of Humor: A Historical Perspective

Another of the complexities in studying the concept of humor is in the style of the comedy itself. A review of the literature of comedy reveals one very striking note: the style of the humor varies tremendously. From Aristophenes to Chaucer, to Moliere, to Shakespeare, to Mark Twain, to Will Rogers, to Joseph Heller and Bob Hope, the range of comedy is almost overwhelming. It is obvious that the social and political climate, the historical events and situation of any particular era or time in history affect the style of the humor. What is viewed as hilarious by one generation may be completely unfunny and not understandable to another.

There are some classic comedies which have survived over the years, but these very often must be interpreted to be appreciated.

> Though comedy has its permanent subject matter and even its
> body of laws, it is liable, like everything else to changes in
> fashion and taste, to differences of sensibility. One genera-

tion's pleasure is the next generation's embarrassment. Much that the Victorians shuddered at merely makes us laugh . . . (Kronenberger, p. 20197).

It is interesting to note, however, that George Meredith, in his famous lecture on comedy in 1877, reflected the thought of the Victorian age when he stated that comedy requires a society of cultivated men and women in a civilization that has some degree of social equality of the sexes!

. . . where they have no social freedom, comedy is absent; where they are household drudges, the form of comedy is primitive . . . . But where women are on the road to an equal footing with men . . . there . . . pure comedy flourishes (p. 210).

Bonamy Dobree (1924) contends that:

. . . in the history of dramatic literature there are some periods labelled as definitely "tragic," others as no less preponderatingly "comic," though of course, both forms exist side by side throughout the ages (p. 202).

Tragedy thrives in periods of great national expansion and power during which values are fixed and positive. In great "comic" periods, values are changing; the times are ones of rapid social readjustment and general instability, when policy is insecure, religion is doubted and being revised, and morality in a state of chaos. However, the greatest names in comedy — Aristophenes, Jonson, and Moliere — flourished in the intermediate periods when tragedy had lost its positive character and men begin to doubt if the old values were, after all, the best.

American humor has had its periods of style and change. The frontier spirit, the need for cunning and strength for survival, and a simple homely philosophy were reflected in our American humor. It started with the exaggerations of the first settlers who came over against the advice of family and friends and were anxious to make good. Exaggeration is the foundation of the wit and humor of Benjamin Franklin, of the tall tales of Paul Bunyan, Davy Crockett, and later, Mark Twain (Harrel, 1962, Nilsen & Nilsen, 1988).

When the western migration spilled over the Alleghenies and beyond, the peculiar brand of humor called Midwestern sprang up.

The Midwestern frontier was a new experience and often a rude shock. Laughter was the only relief. The humor was often "uncouth, boastful, bombastic, and irreverent." It loved to puncture illusions, pretensions of grandeur and snobbishness. The "sucker" or victim of practical jokes became the comic figure from the "tenderfoot" to the "simple soul." The humor enforced social norms, but also, was a method for coping with the hardships and reality. Out of the midwest came a fantastic array of literary humorists; Mark Twain, Booth Tarkington, Damon Runyon, Ring Lardner, and James Thurber. Other comedians and humorists include Will Rogers, Red Skelton, Clifton Webb, Joe E. Brown, Buster Keaton, Harold Lloyd, Jack Benny, Herb Shriner and Bob Hope.

The Roaring Twenties and early Thirties were considered by many to be the Golden Age of Humor. That period spawned such comedians as Charlie Chaplin, Laurel and Hardy, W. C. Fields, and the Marx Brothers.

However, from the Thirties to the Sixties there was a stalemate in this kind of honest healthy humor. People were too stunned by the harsh realities to laugh at their absurdities. This was the time of the depression, war, then assassinations, racial riots and campus revolutions. When you are shooting down the system, it is difficult to laugh at it. The jokes of the period reflected this tension. First there were the empty jokes, the shaggy dog stories, the "Knock-Knock, who's there?", and the elephant jokes. There were also the scapegoat jokes — the Polack jokes, the monster jokes and the sick jokes. Bergan Evans, speaking of the Sixties, called it the age of the "bland leading the bland." He felt people were so insecure they could not bear to be laughed at or to laugh at themselves. It was not a time for satire. Satire, which Evans defines as the "art of being nasty" or the "sword of wit," is a type of humor which is not intended for the masses. Satire is civilized, controlled rage, alien to the popular mind, which expresses its emotions more directly. Pope and Swift wrote for less than one percent of the population, the "literate."

There arose, however, a technique of comedy writing coined by Bruce Jay Friedman as "black humor," a grotesque, absurdist humor similar in many respects to the "gallows" humor described by Freud and the "medical" humor of the health professionals. In times of great stress this macabre, "sick" humor appears in various forms. This particular style of humor will be explored further in the chapter on "medical humor."

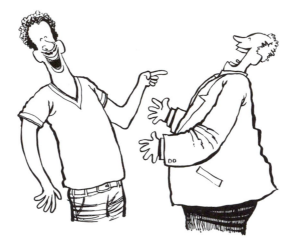

The comedians of the Seventies felt that a new age of humor had begun. One that was honest and reflective and relevant. People were beginning to be able to laugh at themselves again. It was a healthy sign. It was a "renaissance of laughter."

> . . . we have come through the dark '60s craving humor . . . .when you've got that many people angry you've either got to hit, leave, or laugh. We can't leave, and we've tried hitting. Laughter is all that's left (The Denver Post, April 10, 1972).

The new humor was borne in on the waves of "Laugh-in." Satire had a revival. Art Buchwald says the satirist today is blessed with an informed and intelligent audience. Reality is the basis for comedy, and, out of times of tension and turmoil and changing values, arises some of the best humor.

The humor of the '80s is reflected in the rise and increase in the numbers of television situation comedies, comedy shows, comedy in films, comedy clubs, comic strips, political humor, and relevant humor appearing in every popular, scholarly and relevant magazine or journal. It ranges from laughter at our family life to alternate family or single lifestyles, to satire of the society, to a black humor of the sixties. The resurgence of this black humor reflects the stresses of the decade, the conflicting values, the violence and the terrorism. It is reflected in the best selling series, *Truly Tasteless Jokes* and *Gross Jokes*, satirizing every aspect of our society including sex, ethnicity, the handicapped, disease and death! The humor of the '70s and '80s, as seen in the TV sitcom, meets at the center of our culture, says Mintz, and "seems to be more of a compromise, a mixture of warm comedy, simplistic laugh chasing, moralism, and social- topical referencing" (1988,p. 99). A characteristic in American humor, perhaps all humor, is for people to make jokes about things they are "nervous about" (Nilsen & Nilsen, 1988). Certainly, what is happening in any culture or society will be reflected in the humor of that time and period. For a review of the history of humor styles and humor in America, I refer you to Mintz (1988) and Ziv (1988).

# STYLES OF HUMOR
# IN HEALTH AND ILLNESS

Humor about health and illness and health professionals has followed the styles of the era or times also. A book entitled *Wit and Humor of the Age*, written in 1883 by Melville Landon, has a chapter on "Doctors, Wit and Humor." The following reflects the "homespun" quality of that era.

> My doctor, Dr. Hammond, is a great doctor. He can cure cholory or smallpox, or hams or bacon. One day I cut off my toe with an axe. When I called in Dr. Hammond to prescribe for me, he told me to hold out my tongue. He said he thought I had tic doloro, and then he precribed bleeding, and then he bled me out of seventeen dollars. That was the dollar, and when he wanted his pay I told him to charge it, and that was the tic, and I still owe it to him, and that is the "o" (p. 436).

Although medical treatment has changed, complaints about medical fees apparently have not!

The humor of the Forties brought with it the lampooning of the medical and nursing profession, starting with stories and cartoons in the professional journals. The medical student and medical care and the student nurse, the "Probie", were the butt of much humor, and revealed the anxieties of the professional.

> "Quick! Pick it up off the floor before it gets unsterile."
> A student with a tray full of dentures collected from patients,
> says to the head nurse, "Now, what do I do?"

Richard Armour (1963) satirizes the medical profession:

The Doctor's Life
>                Look up noses,
>                    Look down throats,
>                Look up nostrums,
>                    Jot down notes,
>
>                Look up rectums,
>                    Look down ears,
>                Look up patients
>                    In arrears,
>
>                Pull down covers,
>                    Pull up gowns . . . .
>                Life is full of
>                    Ups and downs (p. 3).

The humorous get-well cards, jokes and joke books, novels, and television shows demonstrate that not only is the public more knowledgable about health and disease today, but, also more comfortable in poking fun at it.

A Little Learning

Patients once let surgeons cut
Without an if, or and or but.
They rarely raised demanding questions
And never offered up suggestions.

Patients once, not long ago,
Believed the doctor ought to know,
Submitted with the best of will,
And trusted in his practiced skill.

But patients now, and patients' wives,
Are sharper than a surgeon's knives,
And argue over each incision . . . .
They've seen it all on television (p. 33).

The humor movement of the '70s and '80s has brought forth a plethora of humorous materials about health in the popular domain, and reflects the current research and technology that "laughter is good medicine." A cartoon which appeared in the *Readers Digest* shows a physician on the phone, saying to his patient:

"Take aspirin, drink plenty of liquids, stay in bed and watch an old Laurel and Hardy movie."

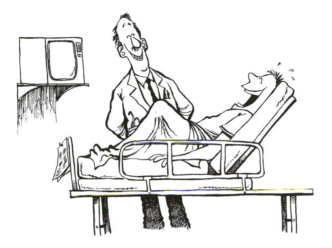

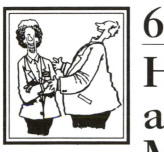

# 6
# Humor As a Healthy Mechanism

The basic assumption or framework upon which this study is built is the belief that humor is a form of human behavior that is healthy and constructive. Yet, despite the recognition that humorous pursuits are a widespread activity in almost all human societies — and the preponderance of authors and investigators who attest to its value — the question of whether humor is healthy or unhealthy continues to arise and that issue is a source of debate (along with all the other issues!).

Over the centuries there have been negative and positive views of humor and laughter from the social and moral stance as well as the psychological and physiological. "For much of Western history, laughter was thought to be impolite at best, sinful at worst" (Goldstein, 1987, p. 3). Only within the last 100 years or so has laughter in public been socially acceptable.

There are still questions raised as to what constitutes healthy humor and laughter from the psychological and the physical perspective. What motivates ridicule, sarcasm, black humor and sick jokes and how does it relate to hostility and denial of reality.

Concern is expressed about the non-humorous, uncontrollable laughter of anxiety and hysteria, the inappropriate laughter of the mentally ill, the cruel laughter at "funny" behavior and deformities, as well as laughter as a result of various diseases, neurological disorders, and lesions of the brain. There is always fear that the use of humor will be abused and be destructive.

That laughter produces healthful results has been supported by armchair theorists over the years, more recently by scientific corroboration. Laughter as an indication of physical pathology is still extensively discussed (Moody, 1978; Duchowny, 1983; Haig, 1988), and each indicates that one must distinguish the healthy laughter from the pathological.

In the mental health field, the controversy also exists. Does laughter reveal health or other problems? Keith-Speigel (1972) points out three possibilities: is the laughing, joking person:

(1) revealing that he is healthy and mentally well-balanced; (2) divulging his innermost hang-ups and deep-seated problems; or (3) is his laughing an indication that he is handling his mental conflicts and worries in a healthy manner by converting them to pleasure?

All three are probably true, and there has been much discussion of each of these areas. There is much support for the emotionally therapeutic value of humor as an adaptive, coping behavior, as a catharsis, as a defense mechanism, as a sign of emotional maturity and as a survival mechanism. But, there are others who have stressed the destructive aspects of humor: producing sadistic, masochistic, guilt and anxiety effects and inappropriate use in psychotherapy.

Freud's concept of joking was based on his original theory of repression and unconscious conflicts. That at which we laugh is indicative of our problems or inhibitions. On the other hand, Freud contends, joking becomes a healthy and socially adaptive way of handling these problems. He goes on to compare humor to other more pathological methods used by humans, namely, neuroses, psychoses, intoxication, etc. Humor, he says, manages the same effect "without overstepping the bounds of mental health" (1923, p. 163).

Martin Grotjahn (1957), in his interpretation of humor and laughter based on Freud's theory, contends that Freud did not go deep enough into the aggressive, hostile aspects of humor. Grotjohn speaks of wit as related to aggression, hostility, and sadism, while humor is related to depression, narcissism, and masochism. He describes the wit, the tease, the kidder, the practical joker, the cynic, the clown as belonging to that large family of people struggling to find a permissable outlet for their aggressions and/or also avoiding depression. A devastating analysis! Yet, he contrasts these characteristics with the statements that "a sense of humor signifies emotional maturity," and "laughter is a sign of strength, freedom, health, beauty, youth, and happiness." There is a need, he says, for this free and episodic regression in order to gain strength for this reality we live in (pp. 255-264).

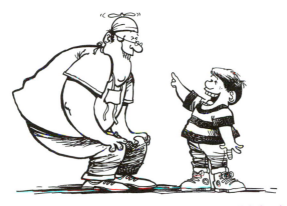

McDougall (1903) describes laughter as a biological instinct devised by nature as an antidote for the depression and pain we feel in sympathizing with the overwhelming misfortunes or miseries of others. It has "survival value." He also describes

> . . . a larger humor which finds occasion for laughter in those defects and shortcomings which are common to all men; such humor including in its object the laugher himself, does not wound, as does the lower, simpler form of laughter; for it brings a bond of fellowship between him who laughs and all his fellows, inviting all men, without discrimination, to share in the genial exercise. Humorous laughter is thus a higher form which implies the attainment in some degree of the power of viewing ourselves objectively, of seeing ourselves as others see us (p. 395).

Moody (1978) discusses at length the pathology of humor from the physical and mental perspectives, and contraindications for the use of humor because of its harmful effects. Yet, he closes on a positive note, encouraging the medical establishment to take itself less seriously! He distinguishes the healthy use of humor from the unhealthy. His differential diagnosis? To be healthy, he says, mirth must occur within the context of understanding, love and support and must include the patient in the laughter.

The results of a 35-year study by Valiant (1977) of a group of healthy men and how they adapted to life indicated that humor was one of the five mature, coping mechanisms these men used. "Humor is one of the truly elegant defenses in the human repertoire. Few would deny that the capacity for humor, like hope, is one of mankind's most potent antidotes for the woes of Pandora's box" (p. 116).

Are these seemingly disparate thoughts contradictions? Or do they merely reinforce again the paradoxical nature of humor and laughter? It is all of these things! Essentially, humor and laughter range on a continuum! There is some validity to each position! Humor is unique to each individual and each situation and must be assessed for its healthy or unhealthy effect.

The very issue of healthy or unhealthy humor is comparable to the problem of defining health and mental health which has occupied the time and concern of health professionals for many years. What is health and what is mental health? How does one know when they have been achieved? Conversely, what is disease or mental illness? The conclusions reached are that health is not merely the absence of disease, but that health and illness range on a continuum and each is a dynamic process of adaptation and adjustment to maintain homeostasis or a balance. Perfect health and perfect mental health are illusions. We have criteria and characteristics for both, but, in reality no one ever achieves that ultimate. Rather, we recognize that health is an individual state and "wellness" is defined in terms of each person maximizing to his own optimal level. This recognition has influenced the therapeutic measures and the professional's role in the achievement of health.

With the advanced research in psychobiology, we have also come to recognize that physical health and mental health are inextricably intertwined. Stress, stemming either internally from within the individual or externally from the environment, can create organic, physiological and biochemical changes within the body. Positive emotions, we are discovering, can also create positive biochemical change.

Humor and laughter, defined on the one hand as a biological physiological reflex and on the other hand as a psychological, adaptive, defense mechanism, share this same phenomenon. Laughter has been described as stimulating positively all the systems of the body, leading to a feeling of well-being. The relief from anxiety and tension which humor can accomplish, dissipates the potentially harmful physiological changes caused by anxiety. Studies have shown that reduction of anxiety prior to surgery has facilitated postoperative recovery and reduced postoperative complications.

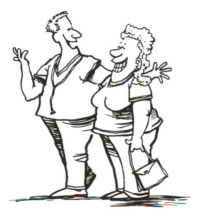

Is not the use of humor as a way of coping with aggression and anger, "health-producing" for the individual? Particularly, if it reduces the rage, hypertension and depression (Fry, 1979). Reik once quipped, "A murderous thought a day keeps the doctor away!" Certainly it must be "health-producing" for the individual toward whom the murderous rage is directed! Konrad Lorenz (1963), in discussing the value of humor, said, "Barking dogs may occasionally bite, but laughing men hardly ever shoot" (p.285). George Mikes (1971) points out that humor keeps man in a sense of proportion, that even though laughter and humor can be aggressive and have a malicious intent, there is reason for cherishing these offensive elements. Human nature, he says, is not peerless and angelic and one needs to get rid of a certain amount of nastiness, so why not laugh it off? Even the most aggressive jokes are better than the least aggressive wars!

In summary, humor ranges on a continuum from healthy to unhealthy. Emotionally, it is healthy when it deals with immediate issues and helps the individual handle realities. It becomes destructive and dysfunctional only when it abets pathological denial of reality — when it becomes a running-away from the difficulties of living rather than an easing of the way to deal with the "heavies" of living.

This aspect of reality-unreality is another issue inherent in this healthy-unhealthy dilemma. The very "play" nature of humor implies a fantasy, an absurd, ludicrous situation which is "not real." This is a joke! Yet, the reality or seriousness of the content of the humor must be evident and intelligible for the listener to "get the point."

Humor is very honest, yet avoids serious implications by placing the comment in a joke frame. Fry (1963) describes the purpose of the "punch line" as projecting the implicit materials within the joke into the "workaday world" of reality (p. 152). Humor, says Lorenz, is the "best of lie-detectors . . . . It discovers with an uncanny flair, the speciousness of contrived ideals and the insincerity of simulated enthusiasm" (p. 287). Thus, humor tends to make the world a more honest place.

Other authors have pointed out that one of the important functions of humor is to relieve us of the burdens of reality. The enjoyment of humor rests upon a make-believe world wherein all the rules of logic, time, place, reality, and proper conduct are suspended. Even sheer nonsense and absurdity are a way to take one's thoughts away from the seriousness of living and provide a feeling that life is not so overwhelmingly tragic. Our sense of humor, Mindess says, "frees us from all the constraints of conventionality, morality, reason and other constrictive forces" (1971, p. 241). The extent of this reality-unreality within each humorous situation, of course, will vary, but it exists as another element in the complexity of humor! Other continuums evidence themselves within this framework of healthy-unhealthy.

There is obviously a range from an immature, more childlike "laughing at" to a more mature "laughing with." Wit, practical jokes, slapstick comedy, the tease, the clown, all fall at the "laughing at" end of the continuum. McDougall's "larger humor," Freud's liberating humor and the humor of the self-actualized man which Abraham Maslow (1970) described as a "humor of the real" and a thoughtful philosophic humor, falls at the "laughing with" end of the continuum.

The functions or purposes or needs which humor serves also range on a continuum from simple nonsense, pleasure to warmth, to social needs, to anxieties, to anger and to the deeper psychological needs around tragedy and death. The kinds of humor and the styles of humor also vary to meet these needs, ranging from nonsense jokes, pleasantries, witticisms to satire and gallows humor.

Within the life and death arena of the health and illness settings these continuums are very evident. Because of the unique nature of this setting, unlike society in general, there are far more instances at the tragedy end of the continuum. It becomes necessary then to look very closely at the use of humor in this context. Whose needs are being met and how? The emotionality of these stresses and tragedies affect the health professionals as well as the patient and his family. If the professional is to use humor as a therapeutic tool, he must be aware of all the issues and the continuums in the nature of humor.

This framework of the nature of humor will be the basis upon which we will explore the uses of humor within health care settings in Section II and the assumptions set forth in Section III in cultivating the use of humor as a therapeutic tool.

# SECTION 2
## HUMOR IN HEALTH AND ILLNESS

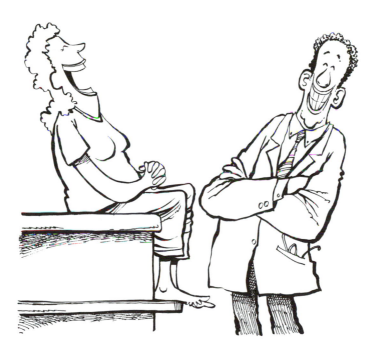

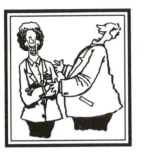

# 7

# Humor in Health Care Settings

Humor is a familiar pattern of communication which both health professionals and patients bring with them into the health care setting. However, humor is not considered to be a formal communication mode. Rather, it is an indirect form of communication, one which is casual and inconspicuously blended into the general flow of events. Because health and illness are "serious" business, humor is not an expected occurrence. Despite this, humor is there and actually occurs in almost any situation.

This "optional" and unexpected quality may be a major contributing factor to the meagerness of studies and descriptions of humor in this setting as well as other natural settings. Of the three major sociological studies which reported observations of humor in hospitals, none was originally designed to study humor specifically as it related to health.

Two studies were serendipitous. Rose Laub Coser (1959) set out to study the social structure of a hospital ward and the role of the patient in it. Her observations of humor and jocular talk led to the formulation of some valuable hypotheses. A second study (Renee

Fox, 1959) was designed to investigate an experimental metabolic ward and the social process of physicians and patients facing uncertainties and unknowns. She discovered that a highly patterned and intricate form of joking and humor was one of the most important ways both physicians and patients evolved for coming to terms with the stresses of facing death.

On the other hand, the third study, conducted by Joan Emerson (1963) was a doctoral dissertation conceived as a step in the systematic investigation of the sociology of humor, but was not concerned with hospitals as such. She chose a general hospital as her natural setting because it was a large organization with a distinct status hierarchy and structured interaction. One of her goals was to show how the nature of humor is related to the structural problems of the setting in which it occurs. She chose two particular "delicate" situations upon which to focus: the pelvic examination and death.

All three provided invaluable insights and contributions to the understanding of humor in health settings and are the basis for this author's study begun in 1965 (Robinson, 1970/78). However, they pointed out the need for more definitive and rigorous investigation. Other studies of humor in health care settings are still meager despite an increase in graduate studies in health disciplines. Humor in health settings has been serendipitous long enough!

# FUNCTIONS OF HUMOR

Within this unique world of health and illness, humor serves three major functions: a communication function, a social function, and a psychological function. Humor serves to communicate important messages, to promote social relations, and to diminish the discomforts and manage the "delicate" situations which occur in this setting. A big order for such an indirect and casual phenomenon! The three functions, of course, are intertwined in any situation. Humor originates internally but requires an audience and must be communicated! Humor serves as a coping mechanism to deal with all the external pressures as well as the internal, intrapyschic stresses related to illness and health care.

# COMMUNICATION

We send messages when we communicate humor with humor. These messages are instant and indirect, but others understand, share our feelings, and they laugh! Sometimes the "message" is simply one of delight, comic relief — a release from reality. But more often, the humor has a more serious message or purpose.

The messages which need to be communicated within the health care settings are usually very serious and emotion-laden: anxiety, fear, frustration, embarrassment, anger, grief, concern, hope and joy. Their direct expression is not always acceptable or comfortable. Humor conveys these feelings in an indirect fashion and, because of its play frame, provides a vehicle for moving easily in or out of the serious as the situation warrants.

In times of illness, strangers (patients and health professionals) are suddenly thrown together, into very intimate and somber contacts. There is no time to build a relationship. The individuals must interact without much knowledge about each other and with no expectancy of a continuing relationship once the immediate health crisis is resolved. The patient must trust the health professional and accept his concern and competency almost on faith. The professional also expects the patient, almost without question, to cooperate with and submit to very intimate, foreboding procedures and treatments and life and death decisions.

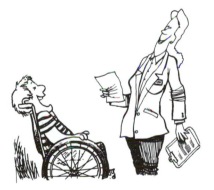

A form of interaction which very quickly provides a sense of familiarity, does not offend, and is easily facilitated, is needed. Humor meets these criteria and is highly suitable for this kind of interaction (Emerson, 1963).

The beauty of humor is that it is in a "joke frame" similar to play: "It's just a joke! It's fun!" Thus, it has a "face-saving" quality. With that little banter, joking, cartoon, or bit of clowning, we deliver a message quickly, without ever having to discuss it and the implicit message behind it.

It can be a message of anxiety, of fear, of anger, of apology, or of embarrassment. It can also be a sharing of a common problem or concern, of warmth, love, support and understanding.

A drawing of a young man pondering this thought:

"Doing a good job here is like wetting your pants in a dark suit . . . . It gives you a warm feeling, but nobody notices!"

And, because of this indirect, "face-saving" joke frame, the listener, even if he does not find the humor particularly funny, will often laugh to be a "good sport." And, if the listener reacts negatively, or does not get the message, the teller can back off with, "I'm only kidding! It was a joke!"

Emerson found that pleasantries around standard topics established the sense of familiarity. This mild form of humor, including banter and jocular talk, provided the flexibility for easily terminating the interaction or for moving into more "serious" humor and a serious discussion. Humor is often used in the health care setting to "test the waters" or as a "trial balloon" to open up to a serious discussion.

The psychiatric patient who kept putting her clothes on backwards was asked why she did. She responded: "Cause I don't know whether I'm coming or going!" A bit of insight!

Dying patient to the staff: "I wish we had pop-up buttons like turkeys, so we'd know when we were done!" Her concern was picked up by staff.

A patient with cancer of the cervix was admitted to the Oncology unit tense, hostile, unable to express her feelings. The physician walked into the room with a 3-foot plastic inflated speculum! The patient burst out laughing and then she began to cry. It broke the ice! He spent the next hour helping her with her feelings and fear of dying.

The humorous comment provides a convenient stepping stone for transmitting more serious concerns. The more highly charged humor with "serious import" could lead to overt discussion if the transition is acceptable (Emerson, 1969). If there is not time or the patient is not ready, it is easy to retreat. However, the laughter or smile of the recipient acknowledges that he has received the implicit message in the joking. Just knowing that others know how you feel is a release in itself, and the fact that the message was conveyed often suffices.

As Fry has said, a joke has a host of unconscious chords which sound in the audience's mind no less loudly than does the explicit joke (1963, p. 67). Joking strengthens bonds between people. By laughing at the same things, we let each other know we share their views without ever having to say so. This is especially true about uncomfortable topics. Both staff and patients bring this kind of communication with them into health care.

# SOCIAL FUNCTIONS

Humor has been called the "oil of society;" it is a great social binder. In health care, it lubricates all those delicate situations and "promotes the continued harmony of a social relation at the same time that important messages are conveyed" (Emerson, 1963, p. 47).

The health care setting is one in which many of the rules of the normal society are disrupted, violated, or suspended. The patient is placed in a dependent role, his privacy is invaded, and the normal social relationships and behavior to which he is accustomed are often waived. Humor provides a mechanism for coping with these disruptive social acts and all the external pressures imposed by the society and the system. It assists in establishing relationships, reduces the social conflicts, provides social control, promotes group solidarity and cohesion, facilitates change and survival in the system.

## Establishing Relationships

Humor is used frequently to establish the relationships which are so vital in the health care setting. It breaks the ice, reduces fear of the unfamiliar, encourages a sense of trust, and initiates a feeling of camaraderie and of friendship. It says to the patient, or colleague or student, "Relax. I'm a friend, you can trust me. This isn't such a terrible place." It sets the tone for a more relaxed atmosphere, much as the main speaker at a dinner will do with his introductory joke or humorous comment.

We make jokes about the environment, the procedures, the instruments, the floppy gown. "Please have one of our designer gowns!"

> When a male patient was sent to a gynecology unit because of
> a shortage of beds, he was teased with "You're in for a
> hysterectomy, of course!"

The patient on admission to this strange and unknown
environment will joke about "all the hotel service" he'll be getting
and all the "pretty nurses to take care of him." Coser (1959/1965),
said "to laugh, or to occasion laughter through humor and wit, is to
invite those present to come closer . . . it aims at decreasing social
distance" (p. 293). She goes on to say that the contribution humor
makes to social economy within the institution of the hospital
should be stressed.

> In such a shifting and threatening milieu, a story well told,
> which in a few minutes, entertains, reassures, conveys
> information, releases tension, and draws people more closely
> together, may have more to contribute than carefully planned
> lectures and discussions toward the security of the frightened
> sick (p. 304).

In this highly structured organization where there is a definite
status hierarchy with the the physician usually as the top authority
figure and the patient at the bottom of the rung, humor also serves as
a leveling agent. It decreases the distance, and is an equalizing force.
Many of the jokes and cartoons about psychiatrists reduce this
all-knowing superior being to the client's level, or at least, to a
human being with a few quirks, too!

> A cartoon pictures a psychiatrist's office. The patient and
> psychiatrist are moving the couch across the room. The
> psychiatrist is saying, "Frankly, Mrs. Watson, I liked the
> furniture the way it was."

In the early days of social psychiatry, during the development of
a community mental health center, in an attempt to move from an
illness orientation to one of "health," and to foster the "blurring of
roles," the staff wore street clothes rather than uniforms. The
clinical director, however, insisted that the staff still wear name
tags, which spelled out: Jane Doe, R.N., and John Brown, M.S.W.
Staff objected that this violated the intent of the change. He

countered that the patients would feel more secure if they knew who the staff were. The controversy ended very suddenly when a day care patient appeared one morning with a name tag which read: Mary Smith, N.U.T. The name tags went the way of the uniforms.

Humor can also establish roles, like who is the patient and who is the professional.

> When a very famous and prominent surgeon became ill and was to be admitted to the hospital as a patient, the staff became quite anxious at the thought of having to care for this authority figure who was used to giving the orders. Finally, one of the nurses drew a stick figure of the typical patient with floppy gown, in flight, with the nurse running after with a hypodermic. She captioned it, "Ha! We've got you now!" and pinned it to the pillow of his bed. When he arrived and saw the note, he burst into laughter! His subsequent sojourn in the hospital went smoothly.

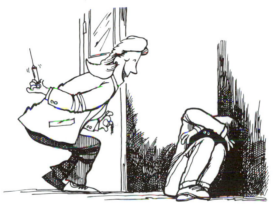

With one small bit of humor, the staff were able to convey their anxiety and concern and remind him of the reversal of roles. With his laughter, he acknowledged his acceptance of the patient role. Within minutes an important message was conveyed that might have taken days and much emotional energy to accomplish.

Humor brings people together. A laugh is the shortest distance between two people, Victor Borge once said. For the patient, if we can laugh a little, things do not seem so bad.

## Coping with Social Conflict

Humor has a way of relieving embarrassment and social conflict. Rules about social conduct and behavior are carefully defined within our society: how we cover our bodies, how and where we perform bodily functions, taboos about touching our bodies, and conventions about the use of certain words in our conversations. Within the health care setting, under the "medical aegis," many of these rules are violated or ignored! Patients are undressed or stripped in an atmosphere similar to Grand Central Station, where all manner of strange persons view their nakedness, where they are poked and prodded, undergo the most intimate of procedures and questioning. However, the rules of the game are that no one (either patient or professional) is to show embarrassment! Rather, each is expected to asssume an air of detachment and nonchalance. Both patients and staff utilize humor to forestall this embarrassment. The humor exaggerates, makes things absurd, and we laugh.

Jokes about exposure, bedpans, enemas, bathrooms, bodily functions and sex abound. The story is told in a number of ways of the succession of males in white, including the painter, who lifts the sheets to examine the female patient. One male patient, in coronary care, who had been systematically exposed, quipped, "I have never felt so naked in my life!"

Performing bodily functions has always been a very private affair in our culture. Whether our bowels moved yesterday is not considered in the same category as the weather as a topic of general conversation (with the exception of TV commercials which discuss "irregularity" with regularity)! Yet, within the health setting, patients are asked to perform on command when specimens are needed; the bedridden patient must be helped and the subject does become one of normal conversation.

On an ambulatory care ward, a patient had signed out to go to the dining room and left a message on the sign board:

> Happy is the patient in the P.M.
>
> Who has had a B.M. in the A.M.

A patient who had had rectal surgery was sent a plant by his friends. It was a cactus planted in a bedpan, with a note saying, "This is one you won't have to sit on!"

Many acronyms and euphemisms have arisen to neutralize this area of conflict. The bathroom is called the "Library." The "throne" is a common expression for the bedpan while the urinal is called the "vase." The uninitiated who are not tuned in to these euphemisms can create situational humor.

> A young student nurse, unaware of the term used for the urinal, hesitated when asked by a patient for a "vase." She looked around a little bewildered and finally asked, "Well, how big is your bouquet?"

Another of the conflicts which face both patients and staff is in the area of the physical examination, particularly of the genital-rectal area. For the female, the pelvic exam is a routine gynecological and obstetrical procedure. Yet it is the "ultimate invasion of privacy that a conscious patient experiences" (Emerson, 1963, p. 167). The discomfort and distaste with which the patient views this procedure has nothing to do with the prospect of pain, but rather with the social attitudes toward touching another's genital and rectal areas. She found in her study that it was usually the staff (most often the male doctor) who initiated the joking around the pelvic examination. It seemed to be "an institutionalized way the staff coaxed the patients to put up with affronts to their dignity" (p. 212). When patients joked, it was usually with the female staff.

Joking about the rectal examinations and procedures occur frequently, both male and female. The awkwardness of the position, the preliminary preparation are occasions for humor. A patient who had had a series of enemas prior to a colonoscopy was asked, "How was it?" She sighed and shook her head and said, "Enemies, enemies, enemies!"

There has always been a high incidence of joking behavior between male patients and female staff. Not only is teasing and joking closely related to flirting and what flirtation can lead to, but in a provocative situation like the health setting where male-female roles are distorted and many of the social rules are suspended, there is confusion and conflict as to appropriate behavior. Many male patients who are placed in this dependent position, who feel powerless, whose body image and masculinity have been threatened, typically respond with sexually oriented joking. This type of humor, in which the patient is relating to the female staff as a man to a women, rather than as patient to professional, asserts his masculinity. If he also makes the female embarrassed and uncomfortable, he asserts his superiority over the situation.

Male patients often tell risque jokes or tease the nurse about "back rubs" and "finishing the bath." A young male patient who had only received a piece of squash for lunch was teased for days by his roommate (in the presence of the nurse) that he had been so excited by the "sweet young student nurse" that he "couldn't even order lunch." A male patient, following a coronary, exercising in cardiac rehabilitation, says to the female therapist, "I've never had to pay so much to see a girl, work so hard, been so sweaty, and never touched her!"

The nurse who may be reacting as a female and does not recognize the patient's behavior as defensive and useful to him at this point, may begin to wonder what she has done to encourage it, and becomes defensive herself. If, however, she recognizes the need behind the humor and responds with banter which diffuses the situation and clarifies her nurturing role rather than the sexual one, she can also use this kind of humor as a cue to other impending threats to his ego.

> Patient: "It's you who makes my heart go pitty-pat and raises my blood pressure!"
>
> Nurse: "Relax. I'm really you're mother-in-law in disguise."

## Promoting Group Cohesion

Promoting group solidarity is a well-known function of humor. Laughter brings people close together. To share common experiences through jocular talk forms a bond and a cohesiveness. Jocular talk differs from a joke in that the humor depends on a knowledge of the actual situation or events and a shared experience. "It unites the group by allowing it to reinterpret together an experience that previously was individual to each (Coser, 1959, p. 301). Within the hospital setting, jokes about the noise and activity ("I'll be glad to get home to get some rest"), poor food, getting "shot like a pin cushion," and nurses who "wake you up to give you sleeping pills," are common. The humorous note reduces the tension, but also serves to socialize patients into the hospital society. Through making light of this culture with all its conflicts, patients adjust to it and cope with it. Their cohesion not only reinforces the hospital structure but through the humor teaches other patients how to adapt to it. The humor also provides a climate for support.

> A psychiatric patient looking out the window at the wooded area surrounding the hospital, quipped, "All the squirrels are on the outside and all the nuts are on the inside!"

The professional groups also have their own set of jokes and joking content which provides for group cohesion and adaptation into a profession and within an establishment in which the same social conflicts are present. The group that laughs together works together! There are the "in" jokes which only the "in" group understands, but which facilitates the group process and the welding of that group.

There is the banter, "Do I have to work with you, again?" or, the adoption of nicknames like "The Sheik" for the surgeon who wears that style head covering. In the operating room, the anesthesiologist is fondly referred to as the "doc who passes gas." Students frequently utilize new terminology or jargon in their joking with each other. During a practice session on the use of the otoscope, the student who had just finished a clinical experience in Obstetrics quipped to the student who was examining her ear, "How many fingers?"

## Social Control

There are so many situations over which we have no control, especially in the health care setting. Humor gives a person or group a sense of control, expresses their feelings, yet maintains the social relationship. Patients make jokes about the rigidity and structure of the hospital environment, the lack of privacy, the laboratory tests and play practical jokes.

Norman Cousins (1979) relates to the constant demand for blood samples and other specimens, and the regularity with which hospital routine takes precedence over the patient's needs. He tells the story of the day his breakfast tray was served along with a specimen bottle for urine. He promptly filled the bottle with apple juice from his tray. When the technician came to collect the bottle, Norman picked it up, held it up to the light and said: "Doesn't this look cloudy? I'll just run it through again!" And, he proceeds to drink it!

Staff also use humor as a way to assert control and convey feelings without destroying the relationships.

> The physician had ordered all stools to be saved on a patient who had been admitted for tests and observation. The nursing staff had disposed of those which were filled with barium and enema returns as not valuable. The doctor, however, quite upset at this decision, rewrote the order to read: "Send everything that emits from the anal canal to the lab." The staff, feeling rebuffed that their judgement had not been accepted, proceeded to send buckets of enema returns to the laboratory and, then, took a large plastic bag used for linen, filled it with air, and labeled it "Fresh Flatus."

The laughter spread throughout the hospital. The physician had to laugh to be a "good sport," but he got the message!

> Cartoon of a patient in bed fully clothed, with suit on and hat. The physician is saying, "Well, well, Mr. Conner, are we ready to go home?"

Humor becomes a "face-saving" device for expressing frustrations, for achieving a sense of control or mastery over the situation and can become an avenue for facilitating change and for survival in this social system.

# PSYCHOLOGICAL FUNCTIONS

In addition to — or concomitant with — all the social stress and conflicts, the patient also faces many intrapsychic stresses and conflicts in the health care setting when illness strikes, hospitalization occurs, and disability and death threaten. Humor often is a major coping mechanism. It relieves anxiety and tension, serves as an outlet for hostility and anger, provides a healthy escape from reality, and lightens all the heaviness related to critical illness, trauma, permanent physical damage, dying and death.

### Relief of Anxiety, Stress and Tension
Anxiety is, perhaps, one of the most common source of discomfort which prompts the use of humor. The "nervous giggle"

is almost a physiological response for some persons. Some authors claim that anxiety is the basic emotion underlying all expression of humor. There is no doubt that it is inherent in many of the situations and overlaps other functions of humor, but it is the prevailing or predominant theme in many instances.

If we look carefully at the current jokes, the humorous greeting cards, and the cartoons, we can detect the anxieties of the times. Approaching middle-age (one never admits that one is already there!) is one of these. A belated birthday card reads, "I'm sorry this card is so late, but I wasn't sure you wanted to be reminded that it was your birthday. Next year, let me know would you rather be old or forgotten?" Another card showing a couple at the breakfast table, the wife staring glumly at the back of the newspaper held by her husband is captioned, "Life begins at forty!" Inside it says, "Begins to what???"

Aging has become a major anxiety in society. Much of the humor relates to the negative — the loss of function, the disabilities — but also to the positive aspects of increasing longevity and health.

> You know you are getting old when:
>
> You're standing at the bottom of the stairs and can't remember if you were going up or coming down!
>
> Your knees buckle, but your belt won't!
>
> You tell your wife you are having an affair and she wants to know who is catering it!

The number of humorous get-well cards, as well as jokes and cartoons about illnesses, hospitals, doctors, psychiatrists and other health professionals, attest to the anxieties related to this area of our society.

> A cartoon shows a hospital room with two patients in bed. One is saying to the other, "Look, you phone down to the desk and ask about my condition, and I'll phone down and ask about you."
>
> A get-well card says, "Remember, it's okay to let your doctor joke with you a little . . . but, don't let him needle you!"

Listen to the joking by patients, it will reveal their latest anxieties and fears. Coser (1959) observed in her study of the hospital ward that the jocular talk related to three areas of anxiety: about the self, about adjustment to a rigid routine, and about submission to a rigid authority structure. The patient is worried about himself, about what is going to happen to him, and is in a strange and unknown environment in which he has lost his autonomy and is faced with a routine and authority structure which increases his anxiety. Humor serves to allay this anxiety. It preserves the self and has a liberating effect. Humor, says Freud (1928), not only has something liberating about it; it has grandeur and elevation. The grandeur lies in the "triumph of narcissism, the victorious assertion of the ego's invulnerability." "The main thing is the intention which humor carries out, whether acting in relation to the self or other people. It means: 'Look! Here is the world, which seems so dangerous! It is nothing but a game for children —just worth making a jest about!'" (p. 6)

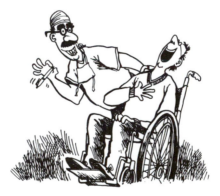

The anxiety about the seriousness of the illness, the procedures, the loss of body parts, changes in body image, permanent disabilities like loss of hearing and blindness, prospects of pain and suffering, and threats of impending death are all areas which precipitate the use of humor.

> A patient who was hemorrhaging quipped: "Is this what you would call a grave situation?"

> A patient being shaved for abdominal surgery, asked the student, as she soaped his chest and abdomen, "How far do you go?" She replied, "As far as possible." As she approached the pubic area, he yelled, "My God, she's going to do possible!"

New technology and new crises in diseases prompt humor in those areas. A cartoon shows a cat with binoculars being held over a patient on a table in X-Ray. The technician is saying, "Relax . . . the first cat scan is always a little scary." When the Herpes and Aids epidemics arose, there was a proliferation of jokes:

> What is the difference between true love and Herpes? Herpes is forever!

> What is the hardest thing about having AIDS? Convincing your mother that you are part Haitian.

Joking and humor is often seen in areas like critical care units, emergency rooms, and operating rooms where the situation is tense, the anxiety for both patients and staff is high, and the possibility of death is a threat. The level of jocular talk and jokes by staff will indicate the level of tension and anxiety. The humor becomes increasingly macabre, risque and gross. There is a need to laugh harder to reduce the increased tension. Sexual, aggressive and gallows humor, areas about which we have the most feelings, will produce the greatest laughter.

When anxiety or tension is too high, reaching panic stage, the humor may fall flat and be inappropriate. According to Freud (1905), "enjoyment of the comic effect cannot emerge unless there is a release of distressing effects" (p. 228). If there is pain or anxiety and the person is himself a victim, all his energy is needed for warding off the danger, and the comic effect is lost. Anxiety must be somewhat controlled before reference to it may be enjoyed in the comic or humorous situation. Only when the immediate crisis has passed or the anxiety has dropped below the panic level will the person be able to laugh. James Thurber once said: "Humor is emotional chaos remembered in tranquility."

Jacob Levine (1950), in a study, found that a joke seems funny only if it arouses anxiety and at the same time relieves it. There are three types of reactions to a joke or humorous happening, he says: if it evokes no anxiety, the listener will be indifferent to the joke; if it evokes anxiety and immediately dispels it, he will find it funny; if it arouses anxiety without dissipating it, he will react with disgust, shame, embarrassment or horror.

When an elderly, dying patient moaned in pain, "Oh God, dear God," an intern stepped behind a screen and said, "This is God. What do you want?" Everyone on the unit reacted with disgust rather than laughter, because for them the anxiety was not relieved, although for the intern it was an unfortunate attempt to relieve his feelings of helplessness in the situation.

Sometimes it is the ludicrous, situational incidents which occur at the height of the anxiety or crisis that provides a "comic relief" which reduces the tension.

> A patient in a critical care unit had not been eating well despite the staff's urging and concern. One day, he suddenly stopped breathing, and, as the nurse, during the code, was pumping his chest, the patient awoke, looked up at her and shouted: "I'll eat! I'll eat!"

> Two staff, struggling to lift a very heavy, embarrassed patient into a wheelchair, watched helplessly, as they stood there holding the patient between them, while the wheelchair rolled slowly across the room.

The humor, of course, is situational, but the absurdity of the event for those who are in it results in the laughter which relieves the tension, embarrassment or anxiety. When we try to tell others who were not there, what happened, they do not find it funny. But, for both patients and staff, this kind of humor becomes a major source of relief for the stresses and anxieties encountered in the health care setting.

### Outlet for Hostility and Anger

The use of humor to express feelings of anger, hostility, and frustration is perhaps one of the most difficult areas for people to accept; yet this is by far one of the most constructive functions of humor.

The outward expression of anger and aggression in our society is generally frowned upon and creates almost as much conflict in our society as sex! But to express hostility through joking is socially acceptable because the target of the hostility can laugh with you. It is a face-saving device. Yet he gets the point. Studies have shown that the enjoyment of aggressive or hostile humor has led to a decrease in hostile feelings. The release of anger in a witty way may do much to prevent the outbreak of hostility or the bottling up of frustration. Humor may also be used to diffuse hostility or aggressive behavior.

Within the health care society there are many causes for anger and frustration. As in society in general, the outward expression of these is usually looked upon with disfavor. Anger at their illnesses, the rigidity of the hospital routines and the dehumanizing elements often leave patients feeling angry and frustrated. To be openly hostile is contrary to the "good" patient role and might alienate the staff upon whom they are relying for care. Therefore, the jocular gripe or joke provides an outlet and performs the function of both complaint and joke. The humor is a safety valve. Comments like "Where else can you get ice water at 5:30 a.m.?" are such evidences of frustration. The patient's anger at his illness is also often revealed and dissipated through the use of humor. One patient referred to his colostomy as "Old Stinky"; another kept calling his chemotherapist "Genghis Khan."

The dehumanizing quality of all the new medical technologies resulted in another patient describing himself as "an extension of the machine." Another patient, alone in an isolation room, put a sign on her door. "If you're afraid of the bugs, at least knock when you go by!"

> A patient who had been sitting much too long in the physician's waiting room, finally was taken into the office. The doctor apologized for the long wait, to which the patient responded: "Well, I did think you'd want to see my disease in its early stages!"
>
> Another elderly gentleman who had been sitting in the waiting room a long time, finally got up and said, "Guess I'll just go home and die a natural death!"

The humor also reflects society's decreasing confidence in the competency of the health professionals, frustration over the increased bureaucracy of the system, and concern about the sky-rocketing costs of health care. Humor facilitates expression yet maintains relationships. "My doctor stops in to see me every day and feels my purse!"

> A cartoon shows a patient clutching a skimpy hospital gown. The nurse is saying, "Well, it covers you more than Medicare will!"
>
> One patient, prior to surgery, gave his doctor a cartoon: Two angels are sitting on a cloud. One is saying to the other, "The last thing I heard was my doctor saying 'Oops!" The patient and his doctor had a warm discussion about his fears!

Humor is often used to deflect and diffuse expressions of hostility and frustration. The angry patient told her Oncologist she had thrown her pills down the toilet. The doctor responded, "Good, now we know the toilet won't get cancer!" A dietician shared a cartoon with a patient who had been complaining about the food:

> Patient: "Is a poached egg too much to ask for?"
>
> Dietician: "Look, you can't expect to eat like a king on a lousy $700 a day.

William Fry (1963) says the relationship between humor, play and fighting may explain the frequent association of aggression and hostility with humor (pp. 101-115).

Children and animals "horse around," wrestle playfully, slap and push and nip at each other, yet never really hurt each other. It is difficult sometimes to distinguish play and fighting — where one stops and the other begins. The participants, however, determine that they are playing, not fighting, and, therefore, there must be meta-communications, cues, and messages which say, "This slap is in fun — not in anger." Therefore there is a "play frame" which says, "this is play — it is not real," although the slap itself is real. This kind of meta-communication occurs in humor and sets a "joke frame." It says, "This is a joke — it is not for real. It is just play." The climax to a joke is called the punch line. "Have you heard this one?" sets the stage for the punch line to which the listener reacts with laughter. In burlesque, it is called the "sock line."

The word "punch" probably originated from Punchinello (a medieval Italian comedy figure), and the Punch and Judy shows, and *Punch* the English humorous weekly. All derive from the Italian word, polcino, for chicken. As Fry says, the cocky rooster, an honored figure in the tradition of comedy, reveals some truths about ourselves as represented by life in a barnyard.

There is also a pecking order to joke telling. The joke teller is the dominant one; the joke is his weapon; his laughter is the sign of victory. The audience is submissive; their laughter is the sign of their acceptance of defeat. "I give up," they say. Then the pecking order gets reversed. "Hey, I've got one!" There are joke orgies in which everyone gets a chance to "punch" it to the others.

Certain figures of speech in our language reveal this aggressive component: "a disarming smile," a "winning smile," "weak with laughter," "a triumphant laugh," "smile when you say that!"

Other authors (Mikes, 1971; Lorenz, 1963) see humor as a way to reduce aggression in our society to a tolerable level. Certainly, both patients and staff can use humor effectively to release bottled-up frustrations and hostility.

Hostile humor is often difficult to accept because it is associated with ridicule and sarcasm. Both hurt and can be destructive. To be healthy, the humor must release the anger without destroying and hurting the other. Humor provides a safety-valve both emotionally and physiologically. Rage and anger dissipate with laughter. They are physiological opposites. Fry (1977) says laughter diminishes skeletal muscle tone and conforms to appeasement behavior so that the body as well is less able to function aggressively.

## Denial of Reality

"And if I laugh at any mortal thing, 'tis that I may not weep."

Lord Byron

Anxiety and anger can also lead to denial. Humor becomes a healthy escape from reality and can ease the way to facing the seriousness and threats of illness and tragedy.

Many instances of humor serve to deny or avoid feelings which are too painful or distressful. The "cut-up" very often falls into this category. He does not stop long enough to allow himself to feel. However, when the stress is too great, this mechanism is one of self-preservation until the person is able emotionally to deal with it. Lazarus (1979, 1984) speaks to the positive effects of denial and illusion in coping with stress. It may be one of the healthiest strategies, especially in the early stages of a crisis, such as a sudden illness, incapacitation or loss, when the situation cannot be faced in its entirety (1984, p. 137). It can lead to hope and then to problem-solving behavior. Freud (1928) has said that unlike other mechanisms for denial of reality, humor does not "over-step the bounds of mental health." In humor, he says, the ego refuses to be distressed by reality, or to let itself suffer. In fact, these traumas are occasions for it to gain pleasure.

When a group of young people were involved in a near fatal accident, the driver of the car called home to tell her parents. The mother, hearing laughter in the background, asked her daughter how they could laugh! She said, "Mother, if we didn't laugh, we couldn't stand all this!" One of the others, who was asleep in the back seat of the car, quipped, "First accident I've ever been in, and I had to sleep through it!"

Many patients use humor to deny the seriousness of their illness. A patient who has received a negative diagnosis may react initially with joking.

> A cardiac patient admitted to the coronary care unit quipped: "The only reason I came here was to get a female roommate!"

> A woman in the emergency room, kept giggling and laughing, as she tried to explain what happened. Her 6-foot son had broken her ribs giving her a bear hug!

When tragedy strikes, humor emerges to help deny the seriousness, and help those involved to cope, especially when there is nothing immediate which can be done to change the situation. It provides a balance and an easing of the way to dealing with the crisis at hand.

The many humorous get-well cards on the market may also be an indication of a denial of feelings. According to Norris (1961-1962), it is a "cover it up with a laugh" or an expression of helplessness even though the person is concerned about the patient. It may be sending a message which says, "I hope you are not really ill; therefore this lighthearted card is appropriate — I hope, I hope, I hope."

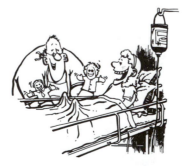

## Coping with Tragedy, Disabilities, Death and Dying

The health care setting is a place where many of the problems from which others in society attempt to insulate themselves must be faced by both patients and staff. In times of tragedy, crisis, disabilities, terminal illnesses, and death, humor is a technique for neutralizing this emotionally charged area and for lightening the heaviness and the seriousness of the situation. The humor does not alter the situation, but provides a perspective and a balance. For that moment, the burden of reality is forgotten; the feeling moves from one of hopelessness to hope. It helps those involved, not just the patient, but the family, friends, and the professional staff to cope emotionally and come to terms with the tragedy and the loss.

Fears about death and dying lead patients to joke about dying and about funerals. The humor helps to open up to a serious discussion and to gain the support, warmth and love they need. Laughing at death helps patients to come to terms with the reality and, as one patient said, to rise above it. The humor and laughter breaks the cycle of despair and frees up the energy used in fearing death to mobilize their own inner resources. Too often the dying patient is treated as though he were already dead. Sharing laughter helps the patient to live until he dies. One patient, hospitalized for recurring cancer, commented that when the staff joked and laughed with him, he knew they cared. It didn't matter what they said, it was the feeling of warmth and caring it conveyed.

Mikes (1971) points out that death is a part of human life, and man has joked about death ever since he was born. The literature is full of funny deaths and funerals. Laughing at death, he says, gives triple pleasure: the pleasure of the joke itelf, the malicious joy of laughing at death's expense and the pleasure of taming death and fraternizing with him (p. 40).

The humor often relates to the discomforts, the symptoms, the pain, or just the absurdity of the situation.

> A patient who was to have surgery for cancer, had been shaved from his neck to his knees. He arrived in the O.R. with his toupee draped over the genital area!

> Another patient who was to have a hysterectomy had written across her abdomen: "No womb in the Inn."

A cancer patient who created cartoons about her experience, joked about the loss of hair following chemotherapy:

> A picture of a bald head with one lone hair sticking straight up, is captioned, "I just washed my hair and I can't do a thing with it."
>
> A group of patients walking in the woods, one is saying to the other, "Don't worry — we can always follow our hair back to camp." (deGaines, 1988)

Comedian Steve Allen, a man who "thinks funny," can "ad lib" at the most stressful, embarrassing times. This facility helped him to cope with surgery for colon cancer (reported in Cope magazine, November 1986). He joked his way through his hospitalization and helped others around him to cope. He recalls kidding the nurses about all the enemas they had to give and thinking of doing a musical sketch about his operation:

> Just after the doctor has removed part of my colon — a semi-colon, or whatever, I suddenly sit up. look into the camera and sing, "All of me, why not take all of me?" (p. 12).

A health professional, who had been hospitalized for elective surgery, had a cardiac arrest in the O.R. She woke up in the Intensive Care unit, not knowing where she was (Heaven or Hell!) with tubes coming out of every orifice including orifices which had not been there before! She heard this voice coming out of the haze, calling her name, and then it said, "We're going to weigh you!!" (New criteria for getting into heaven?)

She giggled throughout the procedure. She said it was the only thing that helped her to survive this stressful situation. Bill Cosby once said that if you can find the absurdity in anything, you can survive it.

Patients with disabling and disfiguring injuries, illnesses and other disabilities often use humor to cope and to put others at ease with joking about their stigma. Geri Jewell, a comedienne who has cerebral palsy, jokes about her disability. She wears a t-shirt inscribed: "I'm not drunk, I've got CP!," and jokes about the number of tickets she has gotten for jaywalking in trying to cross the street. It was her family's sense of humor, creating an environment that told her it was "okay to have CP, and it was okay to fall down," she says, that helped her to accept her disability and encouraged her expression of humor and her career (Goodman, 1989). Humor can indicate a person's acceptance rather than defeat. A therapist knew his group of disabled Vietnam veterans had arrived at a level of adjustment when they began telling amputee jokes.

What do you call a quadraplegic in a swimming pool? Bob!

The type of humor often used in tragic situations is a grim or gallows humor, more macabre, related to the horror, the tragedy and to death itself. The term "gallows" comes from Freud's famous story of the rogue who is being led to the gallows. It was a Monday and the condemned man remarked, "Well, this week's beginning nicely" (1928, p. 161). Although pity is initiated for the condemned man, his stoic jibe saves the person listening the energy needed to suppress the painful emotion of pity. Instead, the listener laughs. In other words, the rogue says: "Don't pity me, laugh with me."

This bravado in the face of death was also described by Renee Fox (1959) in her sociological study of a small metabolic, experimental ward. Because of the gravity of the diseases and the very ill patients with which the physicians had to deal; the constant possibilities of failure and death; the problems of uncertainty; and the trial-and error nature of coping with these uncertainties, a highly patterned and intricate form of humor evolved. As one physician said, "Our humor is a kind of protective device. If we were to talk seriously all the time and act like a bunch of Sir Galahads or something, we just couldn't take all this" (p. 81).

This type of joking seen in this group is so characteristic of physicians, Fox says, that it is generally referred to as "medical humor." In the earliest years of their medical training physicians learn that an effective and appropriate way to handle their reactions to death and other stressful or emotionally provocative situations is to joke with their colleagues about them in a look-it-in-the-face-and-laugh manner. Other health professionals also use such "medical" humor and patients utilize this grim humor to cope with their stresses as well.

Fox found in her study, as did Emerson, that this type of humor rarely crossed the status lines. Staff joked among themselves, but rarely joked with patients or visitors.

However, patients do initiate the humor in this area and there is today more openness and intervention in the grieving process, with more humorous interaction.

> A group of hospice patients developed a bumper sticker which read: "Hospice — what a way to go!"

> A patient recovering from heart surgery, commented, "When you wake up you're convinced you didn't make it, but you're not sure you made it to heaven either!"

An excerpt from a letter written by a patient dying from cancer, just two weeks before her death:

> "I think it is time we let down our hair and told the truth . . . we who are dying of cancer are not martyrs or saints or holy folk. Frankly, if the truth were told, we'd embarrass our friends and we often bore them! . . . I'm still angry about it all, for I think no one has ever loved living more or had more fun doing it than I, and I want it to go on and on. But if I can't, then I must be truthful and say there are a few advantages in living only half a lifetime. Besides the end of good, death also means the end of tribulations — no more holding in the stomach, no more P.T.A., no more putting up the hair in pincurls, no more cub scouts, no more growing old."

Because this end of the continuum, the dealing of tragedy through humor is one which raises the most questions and around which one must look most closely at whose needs are being met, the use of gallows humor by professionals and the role of gallows, black, grim humor in society will be explored in the next chapters.

# SUMMARY

We have described the general functions and uses of humor within the health setting. We will discuss the use of humor for the professional, in various clinical areas, and in education. particularly the education of the health professional.

Humor can heal! Learning how to use it effectively is necessary.

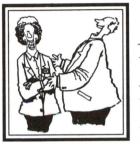

# 8
# Functions of Humor for the Health Professional

The health professional's need for humor is as great as that of the client. Humor has been a major mechanism for coping with the stresses of the professional's education, the "reality shock" experienced in initial clinical experience, as well as the ongoing stresses and hassles of the day-to-day practice of the health professional. Humor serves the same communication, social and psychological functions described for the client. The external pressures and the internal stresses in coping with the professional role are many. In addition to the stresses related to establishing an identity, maintaining collegial and collaborative relationships with other disciplines, and surviving in the health care organization, there are the intrapsychic stresses related to the constant life and death decisions, tragedy, crises, and death and dying.

# SOCIOLOGICAL FUNCTIONS

Humor has been a long-standing occurrence among health professionals. Humor is used to establish and maintain collegial relationships, for group solidarity and team productivity. It is also used for creating change, diffusing resistance to change, and for survival in the health care organization.

Staff use the humor to initiate new members into the organization, making jokes about the setting, the work and the activity. They use joking, practical jokes, banter and teasing for group support and group cohesion and a working together. It reduces the stress and increases productivity. The group that "laughs together, works together." Look at a cohesive working unit and you will find laughter, cartoons, jokes and camaraderie. Each group will have its own "in jokes."

One head nurse of a very busy critical care unit says just throwing out the punch line of their favorite jokes at crucial moments reduces the stress and "keeps them going." Their favorite joke:

> People in hell are being shown various rooms in which to spend the rest of eternity. The last choice was standing up to one's knees in sewage. As one man decided this would be his choice, the devil turned to the group standing in the sewage and shouted, "Coffee break's over. Back on your heads!"

> She also uses "Are we having fun yet?" with both patients and staff in tense situations.

There is also the usual nonsense humor, ludicrous moments, embarrassing incidents, "dumb" student stories and practical jokes which seem non-purposeful, but actually provide the comic relief which reduces the stress and tension. The ability to laugh at ourselves, at our imperfections, is one of the most therapeutic uses of humor:

> A nurse running to a Code, slipped on a wet floor and slid under the patient's bed. She spent the whole Code under the bed, with staff stepping over her head and feet because they did not have time to help her out!

> Medical records sent back to the Unit a number of charts which had been signed off by a very tired night nurse with "Love, Sally."

The "dumb" new student who is sent to Central Supply to get a "fallopian tube," who sprays herself with blood, urine or feces from ineptness, is cause for laughter and teasing!

> In the operating room, the surgeon asked a new student nurse to get him a sterile graduate. The student left the room and came back with "Old Miss Houlihan."

And, there are the usual malapropisms, fractured communications, and slips of the tongue.

> A physician dismissing a large breasted patient with chest congestion said, "That cough syrup should help you. Be sure to return if your chest doesn't get bigger."

> Fractured communications found on patients' charts:

> "Discharge status: Alive, but without permission."

> "Dr. visited this a.m. Expelled flatus. Feeling much better."

> "By the time she was admitted to the hospital, her rapid heart had stopped, and she was feeling much better."

And medical terminology (for the layman):

> Artery . . . . the study of fine paintings.

> Barium . . . . what you do when CPR fails.

> Dilate . . . . to live longer.

> Urine . . . . opposite of "you're out!"

> Varicose veins . . . . veins which are very close together.

Humor within the organization provides a climate of teamwork and closeness and enhances the productivity. One critical care unit reported there were no staff turnovers in seven years and that their climate of "humor" was a factor in the group's productivity and effectiveness. A survey conducted by Abramis (1988) found that the feeling of fun at work is more important than overall job satisfaction in worker's effectiveness. And, a research study (Isen, et al, 1987) found that the elation from humor influenced creativity and improved performance.

Humor is also a powerful tool for creating change and diffusing resistance to change. The bureaucracy and organizational changes can be stressful and disruptive. By laughing at the issues, the frustrations, the absurdities, the silliness of the situation, we can facilitate the change and create reform. Dryden once said, "The purpose of humor is to correct the minor follies of society."

When work hours were computerized in one setting so every minute had to be accounted for, a series of memos satirizing the rigidity of the schedule emerged, including this excerpt from one on "Restroom Abuse."

> . . . . a Restroom Trip Policy (RTP) will be established to provide a consistent method of accounting for each employee's restroom time and ensuring equal treatment of all employees.
>
> . . . . a "Restroom Trip Bank" will be established for each employee. The first day of each month, employees will be given a Restroom Trip Card of twenty (20). Each time an employee uses the restroom, one trip credit will be deducted.
>
> . . . . the entrances to all restrooms are being equipped with Personnel Identification Stations and computer-linked voice print recognition devices. During the next two weeks, each employee must provide two copies of voice prints (one normal and one under stress) to the Personnel Department.
>
> . . . . if an employee's Restroom Trip Bank balance reaches zero, the doors to all restrooms will not unlock for that employee's voice until the first day of the following month.
>
> . . . . in addition, all restroom stalls are being equipped with time paper roll retractors. If the stall is occupied for more than three minutes, an alarm will sound. Thirty seconds after the alarm sounds, the roll of toilet paper in the stall will retract, the toilet will flush, and the stall door will automatically spring open.

Subsequent "memos" laughing at other new restrictions resulted in changes in policy!

When the government imposed DRG's (Diagnostic Related

Groupings) on health care agencies to reduce payments for patient care, agencies began analyzing all hospital and patient procedures for ways to cut costs. Cost effectiveness became an issue and there was constant pressure on staff!

> A cartoon appeared and circulated widely: "Cheer up — we're keeping our charges within the government ceilings!" Pictured were patients on cots in sleeping bags, wooden crates for bedside tables, coke bottles being used for IV's, nurse serving MacDonald's food, physician on roller skates with flashlight skating past patients with tongues protruding and mouths open. Signs posted said: "Help cut our costs," "Play hospital bingo," "Bedpans emptied on Thursday," "Sleeping bags aired first of the month," and "Save your lint for swabs"!

The laughter not only reduced the frustration, but the brainstorming stimulated creativity. We can see all sides of a problem when we do this with humor, and it results in wider solutions. "Any joke that makes you feel good is likely to help you think more broadly and creatively" (Isen, et al, 1987).

Humor can also be a tool in changing values and changing images. Minority groups have long used humor as a way to laugh at stereotypes and to reduce prejudice and discrimination. Within the health care setting, a hierarchy of authority and a role structure exists, with the physician at the top and the patient at the bottom. There is an ongoing struggle for change, particularly in the nurse-doctor relationship. The nurse is fighting to be considered an equal member of the team, moving away from the traditional "handmaiden" image of the nurse who takes order and who dares not make a judgment, while the physician is the "master of the ship" who gives the orders and is infallible! A joke circulating in the system satirizes this "God-like" image.

> A man dies and goes to heaven. He finds a long line at the Pearly Gates and is told by St. Peter that he must go to the end of the line. As he waits impatiently, a man wearing a stethoscope and carrying a black bag goes by and is waved through the gate by St. Peter. The man at the end of the line, rushes up to St. Peter and angrily asks why he let that man in. St. Peter responds, "Oh, that's God. He likes to play doctor!"

A joke not only reflects the social structure and what is going on in a group, but it can rebel against it, seek reform and become an agent for change.

Since a large majority of the health professionals are women, their role in health care has always been influenced by women's traditional roles in society, and subsequently by the change in role initiated by the women's liberation movement. This movement is full of humor!

"Feminist humor is based on the perception that societies have generally been organized as systems of oppression and exploitation and that the largest (but not the only) oppressed group has been the female. . . . it is a humor based on visions of change" (Kaufman & Blakely, 1980, p. 13).

We use our (feminist) humor to deliver our complaints and our frustration because, somehow, we are expected not to offend anyone on our way to liberation.

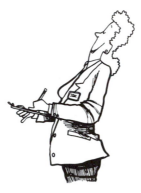

There's an absurd expectation that the women's movement must be the first revolution in history to accomplish it's goals without hurting anyone's feeling!! . . . . curtsey throughout our crusades . . . . smile politely. We've had more than our share of advice on how to be an "acceptable" feminist (Ibid, p. 10).

It is the silliness of it's circumstances that feminist humor satirizes. Feminist humor uses the "Pick-Up" (that is, laughing at itself), rather than the "Put-Down" (which was early hostile humor).

Two women walk into a "Men Only" club. The waiter hurriedly rushes over and says: "I'm sorry, Ladies, we only serve men here." One woman looks up and says, "Good! Bring us two!"

When the "equal pay for equal work" issue was at its height, a cartoon appeared in the health care arena:

A baby girl and baby boy are standing looking down into their diapers. "Oh . . . . that explains the difference in our salaries!"

We can change the image of ourselves or of a group by the humor we use. A sign of maturity is when we can make self-depreciating jokes about the stereotypes, the absurdities, our own problems and deficiencies. And, one indication of any group's "coming of age" in our society is when it allows jokes to be told about itself. Humor can create change.

And, of course, humor becomes a way to survive in the system itself. The organization, just as the family, group, society, or country that cannot laugh at itself is in trouble. In healthy organizations, we see a climate of joking, clowning, cartoons, humorous memos, practical jokes, and playful activities. One director knows that whenever she is out of town, the staff will be arranging some practical joke for her return! The effective manager or leader recognizes the value of humor and utilizes it in practice. A comic perspective leads an organization toward greater awareness of its strength and weaknesses . . . . for new ways to respond and express creativity and to the survival and productivity of its human resources (Jackson, 1985).

# PSYCHOLOGICAL FUNCTIONS: PREVENTION OF BURNOUT

Humor functions concommittently with the external pressures to relieve all the intrapsychic pressures which the professional faces in the day-to-day activities. The humor serves to reduce the anxieties and the stress, becomes an outlet for the frustration and anger, and, is a way to cope with all the heaviness related to critical illnesses, traumas, tragedies, and death and dying.

Health care has become acute care. With all the technological advances in medicine requiring increased skill and knowledge, there are the anxieties about competency and about giving quality care — being overworked and understaffed. There is constant pressure and demands for acute observations, as well as for constant monitoring and critical decisions.

Look at the joking going on in any professional group and it will tell you the latest anxieties, fears and frustrations.

There is a joke making the rounds in the health care system:

> The Pope and the nurse die and go to heaven. St. Peter gives the nurse a white mansion to live in and a white Mercedes-Benz to drive. He gives the Pope a tumbled-down shack to live in and an old pickup truck. When the Pope complained, St. Peter said: "You had your heaven on earth! Remember what the nurse had?"

How do we survive our "hells" on earth? We make jokes and we laugh!

In the areas of the greatest stress — crises, tragedy, critical illnesses and death, the humor of the health professional becomes more macabre — the sick, black, gallows type. It is a major source of coping for staff. It is a way to laugh at the horrors. There is a need to reduce the strain, the seriousness and the feelings of pain, despair and hopelessness which could paralyze and overwhelm the professional and lead to burnout. It is the kind of humor which may seem inappropriate to others, but provides a balance for the individual involved.

> Injured in an industrial accident, the worker's arm had to be amputated at the shoulder. In the emergency room, as the nurse was handed the mangled bloody arm to pack for sending along to the hospital, she noticed the wristwatch was still working! She turned to the others and said: "Wouldn't this make a terrific Timex commercial?"

> In an intensive care unit, three simultaneous code arrests occurred at change of shift. The first patient died. The nurse was wrapping the body as the physician was intubating (bagging) the other two patients. The nurse turned to him and said: "You bag 'em, I'll wrap 'em."

We see the same black, gallows humor surfacing whenever a

tragedy occurs in our society. In 1987, when the Challenger space shuttle exploded, as millions of Americans watched in horror, there followed immediately a rash of jokes and one-liners:

> What does NASA now stand for? "Need another seven astronauts!"
>
> What was the last thing Christa said? "I wonder what this button is for?"
>
> Did you know one astronaut had blue eyes? One blew this way and one blew that way.

One news reporter relating these jokes, said: "Do you know where these come from? They come from us! When we are in the midst of a tragedy, we need somehow to maintain our objectivity, so that we can continue to report and not get overwhelmed by what is happening." We see the same black humor occurring in other professions that are faced with tragic situations — policemen, firemen, the military and, of course, the health professionals!

For the general public, the telling of this black humor has a cathartic effect, the subversion of pain through joking (Zolten, 1987). It is a coping humor as opposed to a hoping humor (Eberhart, 1987). It is a humor that people have always used when they feel hopeless and helpless, when there is nothing we can do to change what has happened. Black humor is a defense against the horror, against whatever it is we fear and is a way to master it, and give us a sense of control by laughing at it.

In health care, this gallows humor is the "medical humor." For the staff, it is a way to distance themselves from the feelings, from the pain, the grief, and the anger, and not to distance themselves from the patient as happens in burnout where the emotions are suppressed. By releasing the feelings through laughter, we can go back to the patient and to giving compassionate care. The black humor does not minimize the situation or provide a solution, but it "transports our spirits" and moves us to get on with the business at hand.

Sometimes the laughing in times of great stress or tragedy is really not funny. It is just a need for leveling, for comic relief. At the end of a long day, we get "slaphappy."! Everything is funny!

Only two students and the charge nurse showed up for work

one day on a 36-bed unit. It was hectic, with patients vomiting and seizures in the midst of trying to give care to all. When the phone rang and admissions announced: "We're sending up two more patients!" all three staff looked at each other, sat down on the floor and broke out in hysterical, helpless laughter!

Sometimes the humor becomes a bit of clowning, joshing, light-hearted banter, a moment of playfulness, squirting each other with syringes of water and "horsing around." In a research study, Coombs & Goldman (1975) found the joking did not interfere with the staff's ability to do a good job, that actually it contributed to the quality of performance because it reduced the emotional strain created by the constant pressure of critically ill patients. Use of humor can be an effective mediator between stresses — even critically ill patients can relax with appropriate humor and the humor becomes a "release valve" for staff in intensive care units (Lieber, 1986; Warner, 1986).

The crucial issue is that this gallows humor may not be appreciated by the patient or the family. There is a fine line where humor does not cross over, even though it is therapeutic for the staff. There is a need to be sensitive to whose needs are being met and the right time and place.

An excerpt from "Reflections" written by an anesthesiologist (Johnston, 1985) poignantly addresses this issue:

> You saw me laugh after your father died.
>
> I was splashing water on my face at a sink midway between the emergency room lobby where you stood and the far green room where his body lay. Someone told a feeble joke and I brayed laughter like a jackass, decorum forgotten until I met your glance over the physician's grey flannel shoulder — your eyes streaming tears.
>
> To you I must have appeared a callous buffoon in green pajamas, a personification of all that is cold and impersonal about hospitals. In silence, I dried my face on paper towels rough as sackcloth, and retreated to the operating room.
>
> My laugh was inappropriate, and for that I apologize. But it was, nonetheless, a necessity . . . . from training and experience we learn to erect emotional defenses . . . . while we may

appear emotionless behind our various masks, please understand: Much of the stress that health care workers suffer comes about because we do care. We cared about your father. . . . All of us worked damn hard. We intubated, oxygenated, monitored, massaged, shocked, injected. And in our own ways, we prayed. Nothing helped . . . . Confronting death as frequently as we do in hospitals causes us to weight the scales with sorrow. We are left to search out our own sources of a counterbalancing joy . . . . the most universal, inexpensive, egalitarian, legal, and portable source of joy is laughter.

Being human, and consequently clumsy jugglers, we will all sooner or later laugh at the wrong time. I hope your father would understand that my laugh meant no disrespect. It was a grab at balance, analogous to what physiologists call a righting reflex — what happens when a cat is thrown into the air.

That day you saw me laugh, I knew that another patient was waiting who needed my care and full attention in surgery. As I stood at that sink and washed sweat and vomitus from my face and arms, my laugh was no less cleansing for me than your tears were for you.

Mea culpa.

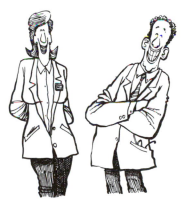

# 9

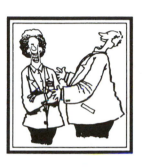

# "Medical" Humor as Gallows Humor

*Man alone suffers so excruciatingly in the world that he was compelled to invent laughter.*

Nietzsche

We have identified the "need" continuum in regard to humor as ranging essentially from simple pleasure to tragedy. We have also established, however, that the need for humor is a very individual phenomenon. How, then, do the two participants — health-care-giver and health-care-receiver — utilize this humor? Is it a mutual exchange or is it mutually exclusive? If the pleasantry, for example, involves only staff who are ignoring the patient, humor can be disconcerting for the patient. However, at the other end of the continuum, if the health professional is attempting to meet his own anxieties about the tragedy which is occurring and if his style of humor does not help the patient who is distressed from a different vantage point (it is happening to him!), humor can be more than simply disconcerting.

Since the style of humor at this end of the continuum is often one of satire or a grim, gallows type of humor — very similar to the black humor style of fiction — we need to compare the styles and techniques and to explore this whole area of the relationship between laughter and tears, comedy and tragedy, and the "gallows" humor to which "medical" humor has been likened.

# COMEDY VERSUS TRAGEDY

This theme or thread tying humor and laughter with tragedy and tears has permeated a majority of the writings on humor. It's an assumption that we laugh so that we may not cry (although sometimes we laugh so hard we do cry!) The relationship is not clearly understood, but its existence is firmly acknowledged. "Man is the only animal that laughs and weeps," says William Hazlitt. "To explain the nature of laughter and tears is to account for the condition of human life" (1819/1960 p. 16).

Koestler (1964) places comedy on a continuum with tragedy, and describes laughter and tears as similar "luxury reflexes" which seem to have no apparent biological purposes but provide a similar obvious relief (p. 31).

Bonamy Dobree distinguishes between three kinds of comedy: "critical" comedy, "free" comedy, and a third comedy which he calls "great" comedy. This comedy is perilously near tragedy and deals with the disillusion of mankind — failures of men to realize their most passionate desires. This comedy makes daily life livable, he says:

> . . . [it] gives us courage to face life without any stand-
> point, we need not view it critically or feel heroically. We
> need only to feel humanly, for comedy shows us life not at
> such a distance that we cannot but regard it coldly, but only so
> far as we may bring to it a ready sympathy freed from terror or
> too overwhelming a measure of pity (p. 205).

This acceptance of "living" is similar in many ways to the acceptance of "death and dying." Kubler-Ross and others have spoken to the need to accept human finiteness and the inevitability of one's own death before the professional can be therapeutic with the dying patient. So, also, the acceptance of human imperfection — and one's own humanness — through comedy and humor manages to assist the individual with the realities of life and living. Humor assists in the retention of hope. If we can joke, things cannot possibly be so bad!

The concept of humor and laughter as a relief from and a way of coping with the realities of life and of dying is an important consideration. Even the "harmless" and "empty" jokes and those of "sheer delight" seem to be a way to avoid emotion, to relieve us of the burdens of reality. When we are immersed in a joke and in the throes of laughter, for that moment, at least, all other thoughts are forgotten. In the life-and-death arena of health and illness, where tragedy and living are highlighted, the role that humor may play in acceptance of both could be vital.

# GALLOWS HUMOR

Freud's basic concept that joking relieves repressed impulses and anxieties, and that laughter converts the unpleasant feelings to pleasant ones, underlies the theory of "gallows humor." This gallows humor, a grim, macabre humor, a bravado in the face of death, is a type of humor which is typically seen when individuals or groups are faced with considerable stress and precarious or dangerous situations, such as at war, on battlefields, in oppressed countries, in concentration camps, and in life-and-death struggles within hospitals.

Obrdlik (1942) describes it as a social phenomenon which has a definite purpose; to ridicule with irony, invectives, and sarcasm in order to become a means of an effective social control. It provides a psychological escape and strengthens the morale of the group at the same time that it undermines the morale of the oppressors.

During the early days of the Nazi movement before the actual invasion of Czechoslovakia, the ridiculing of the Nazi leaders and their regime through jokes and anecdotes was a lighthearted bravado and defiance which gave the people a feeling of security. Although humor temporarily disappeared at the point of invasion when the Czech nation was crushed and bleeding, it was soon heard again. This time, it was more biting, with more irony, and directed at the Czech "traitors" as well.

Obrdlik said,

> People who live in absolute uncertainty of their lives and
> property find a refuge in inventing, repeating and spreading
> through the channels of whispering counter-propaganda,
> anecdotes and jokes about their oppressors . . . they have to
> strengthen their hope because otherwise they could not bear
> the strains to which their nerves are exposed (p. 712).

Some of the stories that made the rounds were:

> Do you know why Hitler has not yet invaded England?
> Because the German officers could not manage to learn in
> time all the English irregular verbs.

> An old man walking up the street, speaking aloud, said: "Adolf
> Hitler is the greatest leader . . . . I would rather work for ten
> Germans than one Czech." When the Gestapo agent asked
> what was his occupation, this Czech admirer of Nazism
> reluctantly confessed that he was a gravedigger (p. 713-714).

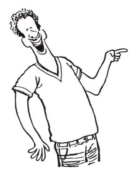

Obrdlik felt that what is true for individuals is also true for whole
nations, namely:

> . . . that the purest type of ironical humor is born out of sad
> experiences accompanied by grief and sorrow. It is spontane-
> ous and deep felt — the very necessity of life which it helps to
> preserve (p. 715).

This type of humor was also seen on the battlefield, by the men
fighting the wars. During World War II, the Bill Mauldin cartoons

and jokes were typical. Willie and his buddy are in a foxhole amidst rubble with bullets flying overhead and he says: "I feel like a fugitive from the law of averages." In another cartoon, the chaplain has been conducting services in the foxhole and he ends with " . . . forever, Amen. Hit the dirt!" (Mauldin, 1971, p. 217-219). During the Vietnam War, a cartoon was produced showing a GI coming through the jungle. A signpost on which Indochina is crossed out and Vietnam is added is attached to a tree. Propped against that tree is a skeleton with a grinning skull clothed in the uniform of a French soldier. The GI is saying, "What's so funny, Monsieur? I'm only trying to find my way" (Mauldin, 1965, p. 110).

# BLACK HUMOR OF FICTION

Black humor (not to be confused with Afro-American humor) has been the subject of much controversy. It has been described as a humor of "grotesque exaggeration, extravagance, sexuality and violence" (Sklar, 1970, p. 28) and seen as typical of American humor from its beginnings. It will continue to express the American character in the future. Max Schulz (1978) calls it an absurdity in existentialist fiction, a divergence from traditional comedy and satire, which "condemns man to a dying world" (p. 7). Bruce Jay Friedman who coined the term black humor suggests that the "chord of absurdity" was struck merely by recording the events of the present age. The satirist had to go beyond satire because his ground had been usurped by the newspaper reporter. Finally, black humor has been defined as a "bitter emphasis on the absurd that makes us laugh so that we will not cry." Joseph Heller, who wrote the classic *Catch-22*, once said that he wanted people to laugh and then look back in horror at what they were laughing at (1971).

When the world could no longer avoid or deny the emotionality of the grim prospects of death, of racial tensions, threats to establishments and changing sexual mores, and when the empty, bland, harmless humor of the Fifties no longer sufficed, the grotesque absurdist fiction of black humor arose. It was a move to the opposite extreme: "making fun of," in the most grotesque, macabre manners, those very things which frightened and disturbed society. It seemed to be almost an attempt to "shock" ourselves out of the horror and anxiety. If we shout the four-letter words often enough, detail the most intimate sexual experience often enough, revel in the most macabre aspects of illness and death often enough, relate the lurid aspects of war and riot and killings often enough, soon they become commonplace, meaningless and emotionless.

In black humor, death and illness and disease and bodily injury are dealt with in a similar, macabre way although through the eyes of the lay person rather than the professional. In the two classics, *Catch-22* and *One Flew Over the Cuckoo's Nest*, the whole medical system is satirized. From the perspective of the patient, fears, horrors, and anxieties about illness and death are grotesquely revealed as well as the incompetencies of the health professionals and the corruptness and dehumanizing quality of the health system.

*Catch-22* revolves around the fear of death felt by the chief character, Yossarian, and his attempts to avoid the bombing missions and stay alive.

> Yossarian was a lead bombardier who had been demoted because he no longer gave a damn whether he missed or not. He had decided to live forever or die in the attempt and his only mission each time he went up was to come down alive (Heller, 1955, p. 30).

Yossarian's thoughts about death are thrust at the reader again and again.

> . . . a placid blue sea . . . that could gulp down a person with a cramp in the twinkling of an eye and ship him back to shore three days later, all charges paid, bloated, blue and putrescent, water draining out through both cold nostrils (Ibid, p. 18).

> People knew a lot more about dying inside the hospital and made a much neater, more orderly job of it. They couldn't dominate Death inside the hospital, but they certainly made her behave. They had taught her manners . . . .There was none of that crude, ugly ostentation about dying that was so common outside the hospital . . . People didn't stick their heads in ovens with the gas on, jump in front of subway trains or come plummeting like dead weights out of hotel windows with a whoosh! Accelerating at the rate of thirty-two feet per second to land with a hideous plop! on the sidewalk and die disgustingly there in public like an alpaca sack full of hairy strawberry ice cream, bleeding, pink toes awry (Ibid, p. 170-171).

The whole crazy medical system, which Yossarian looks for help to avoid flying by his frequent visits to the hospital, is also satirized. The physician, Doc Daneeka, is an absurd figure who:

> . . . brooded over his health continually and went almost daily to the medical tent to have his temperature taken by one of the two enlisted men there who ran things for him practically on their own, and ran it so efficiently that he was left with little else to do but sit in the sunlight with his stuffed nose and wonder what other people were so worried about (Ibid, p. 33).

The two enlisted men, Gus and Wes,

> . . . succeeded in elevating medicine to exact science. All men . . . with temperatures above 102° were rushed to the hospital. All those except Yossarian . . . with temperatures below 102° had their gums and toes painted with Gentian Violet solution and were given a laxative to throw away into the bushes (Ibid, p. 31).

Of course, the "soldier in white, who could not have been any sicker without being dead," is the epitome of the grotesque. Encased from head to toe in plaster and gauze with only an empty dark hole over his mouth, and all four limbs hoisted in the air by cable and weights, he is fed by his own wastes.

> A silent zinc pipe rose from the cement on his groin and was coupled to a slim rubber hose that carried waste from his kidneys and dripped it efficiently into a clear, stoppered jar on the floor. When the jar was full, the jar feeding his elbow was empty; and the two were simply switched so that stuff could drip into him (Ibid, p. 10).

The "mechanical encrusted on the living" is vividly displayed in the reaction to the soldier who was "more like a stuffed and sterilized mummy. Nurse Duckett and Nurse Cramer kept him spic and span." They brushed his bandages with a whiskbroom, scrubbed the casts, polished the pipes and glass jars. "They were proud of their homework." Yossarian and the other patients wonder if he can hear; if he's breathing if it never moves; and, if it's a he! Yossarian finally asks the nurse, "How the hell do you know he's even in there?"

In Kesey's *One Flew Over the Cuckoo's Nest* (1962), the psychiatric hospital is satirized in all its bizarreness, portraying the often-held theme that the society within the hospital is "kookier" than that outside its walls, and that the so-called "therapeutic" measures only tend to reinforce the problems with which the patient enters the hospital. The big nurse, the impotent psychiatrist, and the sadistic attendants are the epitomes of all the patients' worst fears. McMurphy tries to bring some reason and normalcy into the system and we revel in all his rebellious escapades and antics. Humor and laughter is the key to the changes which he creates. He finds the patients are "scared to open up and laugh."

> You know, that's the first thing that got me about this place, that there wasn't anybody laughing. I haven't heard a real laugh since I came through the door, do you know that? Man, when you lose your laugh, you lose your footing. A man go around lettin' a woman whup him down till he can't laugh anymore, and he loses one of the biggest edges he's got on his side (Ibid p. 65-66).

The change to the ability to use laughter is revealed in how the patients manage the uncomfortable, embarrassing situation of being sprayed for lice after their return from their boat trip.

> We lined up nude against the tile, and here one black boy came, a black plastic tube in his hand, squirting a stinking salve thick and sticky as egg white. In the hair first, then turn around an' bend over an' spread your cheeks!
>
> The guys complained and kidded and joked about it, trying not to look at one another or those floating slate masks working down the line behind the tubes, like nightmare faces in negative, sighting down soft, squeezy nightmare gunbarrels. They kidded the black boys by saying things like "Hey, Washington, what do you fellas do for fun the other sixteen hours?" "Hey, Williams, can you tell me what I had for breakfast?"
>
> Everybody laughed. The black boys clenched their jaws and didn't answer; this wasn't the way things used to be before that damned redhead came around.
>
> When Fredrickson spread his cheeks there was such a sound I thought the last black boy'd be blown clear off his feet.

"Hark!" Harding said, cupping his hand to his ear, "The lovely voice of an angel" (Ibid, p. 227).

The laughing and obscene comments served the patients' needs for covering up their embarrassment and humiliation although the attendants did not find it funny.

Ziv (1984) calls black humor a defense mechanism, not only dealing with death, but with all subjects that arouse fear in general. This black humor (or horror humor, sick humor, grim humor or gallows humor) defends rather than surrenders, and masters the fear, like "whistling in the dark." "The opportunity that we are given to laugh at things that are basically frightening or sad protects our mental health" (p. 58).

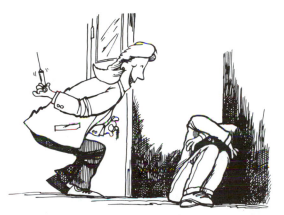

## PATIENTS' USE OF GALLOWS HUMOR IN THE REAL SETTING

Within the real hospital setting, patients have been observed using similar gallows type humor to cope with stressful situations.

During the second World War, on a ward of returned combat soldiers who were both amputees and blind, the use of humor was observed by this author as a frequent form of expression by the men. Many of the patients were fitted with artificial eyes which had to be removed and the eye socket cleaned several times a day during the adjustment period. The workmanship was so fine that it was often difficult for the nurse to tell the difference and would have to ask the patient. Frequently, he would point to the wrong one or squeeze the eye so that it dropped out and laugh hilariously at the nurse's shock and dismay. When patients walking down the hall on the center rubber runner, which was their guide, bumped into each other or into staff, the common response was, "What's the matter with you? Got eye trouble?"

In the experimental metabolic ward studied by Renee Fox, the use of humor was one of the ways patients came to terms with the problems and stresses they shared. They joked about their inactivity, incapacity and isolation. They made jokes about the experimental surgery, the drugs, and their roles as human subjects. They wrote medical documents satirizing a "case history" and a "report of death" with such statements as, "He died 'cause he was too damn lazy to live." Much of the joking revolved around the way they were subject to the medical program.

> I think the reason I'm so fouled up is because of all the gooey stuff they're always sticking in my veins. My veins must be coated an inch thick with all that sticky albumin and resin. What I need is an I.V. of Sani-Flush.

They designed a coat of arms for the ward: two crisscrossed hypodermic needles, with a drop of blood suspended from the tip of each.

Finally, there were "death" jokes. These were the most "frequently made and the most relished" (p. 173). "I sure came close to the pearly gates, all right! I knocked on them, but Saint Peter told me to get the hell out!" They played at summoning up spirits who came back to haunt those still alive. A patient, reacting to a group of doctors discussing his case at his bedside, joked, "You fellows better get it together quick . . . can't you see I'm dying?"

"Laughing at their hopes about getting well, made it easier for them to come to terms with the fact that, actually, this might never be possible" (p. 176).

## "MEDICAL" HUMOR

Similarly, the hospital and its medical staff must deal with these problems and fears, the ultimate being death with all the degrees and potentialities of that: minor illness to critical illness to disability and disfigurement. The handling of the body and all the intimate procedures which have sexual implications is another area of conflict in our society.

The type of laughing-at-death gallows humor which Renee Fox called typical "medical" humor has been used by all health professionals in adjusting to the "reality shocks" of their chosen occupations.

Student nurses and medical students give fond names to cadavers, either human or animal, that they use to study anatomy and physiology. A favorite jingle when tuberculosis sanitariums still flourished was:

> T.B. or not T.B.,
>
> That is congestion,
>
> Consumption be done about it?
>
> Of corpse! Of corpse!

Death and the procedure for preparing the body for the morgue often provoke a "laughing at death" approach. On one occasion, when an old gentleman had died, the two student nurses who were on duty that night prepared the body for the morgue in the absence of the orderly. They straightened the limbs and gently but securely tied them with gauze bandages. Then, discovering that the "sexual appendage" was erect, gaily decorated it with a huge gauze bow, brightly dotted with red and blue ink.

The frequent association of food to blood and viscera is common:

> Liver again! Pathology must have had an oversupply this week!

In the operating room and emergency room, where tension is the highest, humor becomes almost a standard pattern of interaction, from simple, jocular talk to macabre, risque joking.

> Two students were observing surgery for the first time. The shorter one was complaining she couldn't see. The tall one quipped, "Be glad you're not tall. You have a longer way to fall when you faint!"

> During an operation, the assisting doctor told a joke: "Do you know what happened to the nurse who swallowed a razor blade? She performed a tonsillectomy, a hysterectomy, and circumcised an intern."

Renee Fox describes the form of "gallows humor" which the physicians used on the experimental metabolic ward she studied. They joked about the uncertainties, their inability to "cure" patients and some of the impending deaths; they made bets about the unknown. This freeing of tension helped them to come to terms with their situation in a useful and professionally acceptable way.

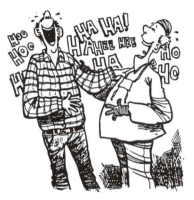

Dr. D.: Mr. Goss is still alive.

Dr. S.: Is he putting out urine?

Dr. D.: No.

Dr. E.: Is he having hemodialysis?

Dr. D.: No.

Dr. C.: Then how is he alive? (laughter)

Dr. C.: I'll give you 10 to 1 that Mr. Green had Addison's disease.

Dr. D.: I won't take it . . .

# GALLOWS HUMOR: WHOSE NEEDS ARE BEING MET?

The significant consideration at this point must be whether or not the gallows type of humor used by patients and by staff with their peers is appropriate to be cultivated by staff to use in interaction with patients. Sociologist Coser has suggested that humor across status lines may well take other forms and have other functions that humor among status equals. In discussing the possitive effect of gallows humor, Obrdlik also speaks to the negative effect, a disintegrating influence among those against whom it is directed. "The black humorist," Hamlin Hill contends, "does not seek the sympathy or alliance of his audience, but deliberately insults and alienates it." It becomes a moot question then, since gallows humor appears to relieve one's own anxiety, not necessarily those of others. This is particularly true when the other may be the object of the tragedy.

The medical humor generally used by the health professional has always been to support his own needs, to relieve his own anxieties and concerns, and to avoid those aspects of tragedy which he is expected to play a large part in preventing by his skills and knowledge. The paradox is that the medical humor brings him closer to his colleagues, to share in the realization that he is not a hero, is not perfect, is still human. Yet the patient is depending upon him to prevent death, to avoid disability, and to cure his illness. He is expecting and paying for seriousness, for miracles, and for godliness.

Emerson states that more watchfulness is necessary in regard to humor than in most matters because by its very nature, humor is always toeing the line between divergence and defiance, tettering on the verge of going too far.

In the television series "M*A*S*H," this fine line seemed to be achieved. They demonstrate very clearly the staff's need for humor as a way to survive, yet in no way do they put down, depreciate, or laugh at the patient. The staff still maintains that quality of concern, caring and competency despite their zaniness. The health professional is always in a dilemma of having to appear as the all-knowing, miracle-worker with a god-like air to meet patients' expectations. Yet underneath, the professional knows he is as human and vulnerable as the rest.

The humor between colleagues is very often a self-depreciating one which is acceptable within status lines, but might not be understood in the same vein by the patient. This story making the rounds some years ago may serve as an example.

> Two psychiatrists are coming down in the elevator after a
> day in the office. The younger psychiatrist looks weary and

somber. The older psychiatrist is whistling cheerfully. The younger man looks over and says,'How can you be so spry and cheerful after a long day of listening to patients with all their problems and troubles?' The older man shrugs his shoulders and responds, "Who listens?"

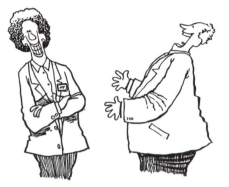

This may tickle the fantasies of the psychiatric staff, but might be very threatening to the patient who will always wonder if his psychiatrist is really listening.

Much more research in needed in the area of gallows humor. It may very well be that its use is a limited one for medical professionals with patients. However, the value and usefulness of gallows humor for patients and staff as a mechanism for coping cannot be overlooked, and therefore, should not be discarded. The recognition of whose needs are being met and when and in what situation seems to be the crucial factor. The fine line or delicate balance between use by staff and use by patients must be found. There may be times when a gallows-type humor may be appropriate across status lines in the right situation and the right time.

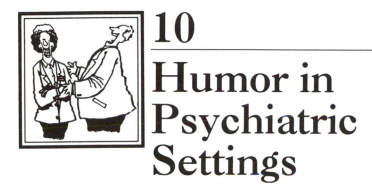

# 10
# Humor in Psychiatric Settings

Traditionally, we have laughed at the "crazy" behavior of the mentally ill person. Many jokes, cartoons, and comedies revolve around and mimic this abnormal behavior. The professional who works with emotionally disturbed persons often justifies his laughter as the only way he can keep his own sanity. Traditionally, however, this disparaging laughter never occurs in the presence of the patient. Rather, the "seriousness" of the situation and the "mental state" of the patient has usually precluded the use of humor as appropriate in the treatment or therapy of the psychiatric patient.

The use of humor in psychotherapy, in counseling and in group therapy has been controversial. Early on, most of the objections came from the classical psychoanalysts, which is surprising since it was Freud who pioneered in this area of humor. The lack of focus on humor as a factor in therapy and the present controversial opinions may very well have been the result of Freud concentrating on the hostile wit rather than the mature, empathetic humor (O'Connell, 1976).

Freud has been described as a story teller and lover of jokes who used his patient's jokes and dreams in his therapy. Alfred Adler was also described as having an abundance of humor. Adlerian psycho-therapy, which emphasizes encouragement as a primary technique and keeping the patient's hope elevated as one factor in this technique, suggests that humor assists in the retention of this hope.

Other analysts have suggested that eliciting from patients their favorite jokes could be useful in revealing anxiety around areas of conflict and repression. Zwerling (1955) points out that this technique may lead lightly and naturally into discussions of such areas of conflict and may be particularly useful when a light touch is needed for a tentative approach to a troubled area. This technique offers insights in the same way as dreams, memories, and responses to projective techniques, but has the advantage of being more concise and pointed. However, this technique has several limitations, Zwerling says, which are valuable points to be considered. Some patients fail to have a favorite joke and some patients may resort to the latest joke they heard. The "favorite joke" may also be a learned one, that is, told with repeated success several times so that it achieves the status of favorite joke, but does not bear any relationship to the problems of the teller. Other limitations may be that the joke may reflect the social problems of the patient's particular culture, but may not necessarily represent his specific conflict. Or, a patient's neurosis may be so complex that a great variety of jokes would reflect some aspect of his personality. However, he says, this technique should be useful in any system of therapy that recognizes the personality as a unit in which every part is related to the whole.

In contrast, and adding to the controversy, Morris Brody (1950) maintained that laughter was not common during the analytic hour except as a reaction to occasional wit, and, as a rule, it is the sickest type of personalities (the schizophrenic, schizoid or compulsive) who smiles or laughs during the analytic session. The analyst may call attention to his laughter, but once this happens, the patient becomes uneasy, fearing he is being laughed at or accused of having laughed at the analyst. Laughter, Brody says, is a defense best left undisturbed because the meaning of the laughter is too buried in the unconscious.

Nussbaum and Michaux (1963) explain that the schizophrenic's inability to experience humor is a result of his conceptual disorganization which interferes with his "getting the point of a joke" but that the patient with an affective disorder will at least intellectually understand it. The inability of the depressed patient to react to humor may be due to a "freeze of affect:" if it is certain that he has not been too preoccupied to listen to the joke and to understand it. On this assumption, then, the reaction of the depressed patient to humor could be utilized as a predictor of the course of the illness. As the depression lifts, his ability to react to humor may improve. The results of experimental study by Nussbaum and Michaux offered tentative support to this theory. They found reactive depressives responded better than psychotic depressives with grandiose guilt feelings, but that in patients with schizophrenic overtones, the schizophrenic ideation increased.

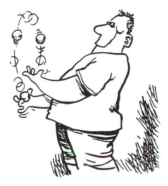

In a situation observed by this author, a patient who became depressed following gallbladder surgery demonstrated this increased response to humor as her depression lifted. It had been noted, however, that the patient had often used humor as her pattern of interaction prior to surgery. The nursing staff in their plan for nursing care utilized humor as an approach to intervening in the depressive reaction with subsequent positive results (Robinson, 1970, 1978).

The use of humor as a deliberate technique by an analyst in individual therapy has been an ongoing discussion with many controversial feelings. Lawrence Kubie (1971) warned that humor has a high potential for destructiveness, that it can be a dangerous weapon, and the mere fact that it amuses and entertains the therapist and gives him a pleasant feeling is not evidence that it is a valuable experience for the patient. His intent, Kubie says, is not to persuade us never to use humor or that it is always destructive, but that this potential should be considered. Humor can be a humanizing influence, ease tension in social situations, and express true warmth and affection, but it is also used to mask hostility and, in the hands of an anxious or junior analyst, can be harmful. Kubie then points out some significant considerations in the use of humor.

Although humor may facilitate the flow of free associations, it may block or arrest the patient's spontaneous stream of thought and may also confuse the patient as to whether the therapist is serious or "only joking." Humor can be used by the analyst as a defense against his own or the patient's anxiety and as a mask for his own hostility. The patient may feel compelled to join in the humor "to be a good sport," thus finding it impossible to express anger or resentment. If the patient uses self-depreciating humor and the therapist joins in, this may deepen the patient's self-depreciating feelings.

Patients also may use humor as a defense against accepting the importance of their own illness. If we laugh, we may reinforce this defense. A gentle, sympathetic humor can be used more appropriately when the treatment process seems to be approaching a successful termination; as one of the signs of improvement, or to mobilize new insight, Kubie concludes.

The critical issue is that it is never justifiable to make fun of or to laugh at the patient or his symptoms. Laughing with someone rarely does harm. How to make this distinction may be the most difficult decision in the helping process. In the hands of a senior therapist, Kubie says, humor at such times can be a safe and effective tool. In the hands of a new, inexperienced analyst who may be imitating the senior too early in the game, it may not. Humor, Kubie contends, also impairs the therapist's necessary "incognito" — the doctor sitting silently behind the patient laying on the couch, distant and detached, and failing to establish a social relationship with the patient, or sharing of the analyst's personal life or experiences. The psychotherapeutic relationship is a highly charged one and puts a demand on the psychotherapist for a degree of wisdom and maturity man has not reached, Kubie says. This technical device places a distance between patient and doctor and serves to protect the patient from the frailities of the therapist. Humor, he says, "has its place in life. Let's keep it there."

The question is: what is its place in life? Is not psychotherapy dealing with the problems of life and the patient's living in it? Mindess (1971) makes a cogent statement:

The point is that to encourage a humorous outlook in his patients the therapist must keep the dimension alive in himself. If he can perceive the irony in their predicaments and in his own as well, his perception will permeate his interviews and will, when his patients are supple enough to take it, enlarge their comprehension of themselves.

But there's — I'm afraid we must confess — the rub. A glance at any professional journal, or a visit to any professional meeting, makes it apparent that psychotherapists take themselves too seriously. We really believe — and the more renowned among us believe it the more — that the theories we propound and the techniques we apply are cogent, valid, and beneficial. Not only do we believe it; we must believe it to be effective. And yet, as long as the belief is maintained, a deep and genuine sense of humor cannot be achieved and therefore promoted. As long as we fail to contemplate the likelihood that our professional activities are useless — that psychotherapy of any sort is absurd in the larger scale of things — we remain bound to the very outlook from which we need to free our patients (p. 220).

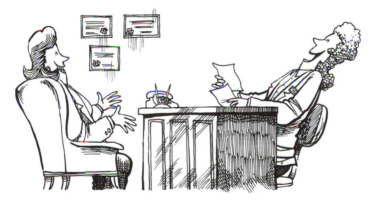

Mindess (1976) further proposes that "a humorous assessment of life can cut deep; it can expose hidden truths and articulate philosophical positions of no little moment . . . . I have seen people cope with problems small and great by perceiving their ironic dimensions. I have also seen people come to terms with themselves, in part at least, by perceiving their own absurdity" (p. 334).

Another analyst, Warren Poland (1971), also reacts negatively to Kubie with the belief that humor can be constructive in psychotherapy and that the incognito technique was devised not to serve as a defense for the analyst, but to frustrate the patient's wish for transference gratification and should be used only to the extent it promotes further psychologic work by the patient. Before using humor, Poland says, the therapist should evaluate the strength of the therapeutic alliance. When humor is integrated, appropriate, and spontaneous, it is indicative of a good therapeutic alliance and informative of the presence of the patient's observing ego. To refute Kubie's statement that therapists never reveal their use of humor, Poland cites two cases.

In one example, a patient's initial response to the relationship was one of enthusiasm, pleased at everything the analyst had to say. After about two months, this changed to the opposite, with the patient complaining about the analyst, no matter what he did or said:

> At one point in the patient's discourse . . . he reflected, "I used to hang on your every word." With a laugh [the analyst] spontaneously erupted, "And now I hang on my every word."

The patient laughed and was able to use this interpretation to look at the process.

Another analyst, Gilbert Rose (1969), analyzed humor and pointed out how it may operate beneficially in treatment. First, he says, humor depends on the analyst's personal style. Second, the analyst, having a talent for the use of humor, depends on his tact, judgment, and awareness in weighing the effects of the humor at a given moment. Third, the use of humor should always be directed toward a stable therapeutic alliance. Used in this way, Rose says, humor is not an evasion of reality, but an invitation to collaborate to increase awareness. He analyzes specific benefits. Humor may be used to mobilize benign aspects of the superego and support the ego. It may be used to lift repression and render acceptable an interpretation that otherwise cannot be made. It may transmit reality in the right blend of closeness and distance. He gives several examples: The remark to a patient, "If you go on like this, I may have to believe in the unconscious," makes use of the mechanism of negation to convey several interpretations. Light humor may be one way to interpret a sexualized transference resistance. "I'll bet you say that to all your psychiatrists," is an appreciative response to a patient's seductive communication, a recognition that it is just a "line," but the work of treatment will go on. Humor, Rose feels, may play a part in establishing and maintaining a freer interaction between patient and analyst.

This freer interaction and the more open, sharing, reality-oriented approach to the care and treatment of emotionally distressed individuals is reflected in most of the other psychotherapeutic models in recent years. It not only reflects the acceptance of humor as a reality of life and as an integral part of the communication pattern between patient and therapist, and between patient and patient, but also reflects the patient's ability to laugh at himself. "The neurotic who learns to laugh at himself may be on the way to self-management, perhaps to cure. (Allport, 1950, p. 92) humanistic and existential psychotherapies reflect this philosophy.

Viktor Frankl (1963) incorporated humor in his method of therapy called logotherapy. As a student of Freud, he began his career with a psychoanalytic orientation, but became influenced by the writings of existential philosophers. His philosophy and therapy were tested and strengthened by his experience as a prisoner in a German concentration camp. Frankl found that man can preserve a vestige of spiritual freedom even in such terrible conditions. If there is a meaning to life, there is a meaning to suffering. This will to find meaning is the basic concept of his therapeutic process. His aim is to enable the patient to acquire a new perspective, to rise above the powerful negative driving forces in his life and to a new and true meaning in life. One's sense of self is not seen as fixed but rather one's sense of self is laughed at for its foolish and self-defeating strivings. Humor as the capacity to laugh at oneself is a natural characteristic. This quality of self-detachment in humor is utilized in a procedure Frankl calls paradoxical intention. It is based on the concept that what one fears happens, but hyper-intention makes impossible what one wishes. As soon as the patient stops fighting his obsessions or phobias and starts ridiculing or joking about them, the vicious circle is cut and the symptom diminishes and atrophies.

Other professionals in the field of mental health have also pursued the positive approach to the role of humor in psychotherapy with techniques applicable to individual and group therapy, and in the milieu of the psychiatric in-patient setting. Humor is not restricted to any specific theoretical framework. Many therapists who are humorously endowed use humor naturally in their daily work, other therapists have made humor their cornerstone and have developed theories of psychotherapy built around it (Salameh, 1983).

Walter O'Connell (1976, 1981, 1987) calls his approach "natural high" therapy. It is based primarily on Adlerian theory and humanistic philosophy. The therapeutic goals are self-esteem and social interest. The client's sense of humor is fostered in the self-actualization process — a "natural high." The therapist models the humorous attitude by self-depreciating humor. This approach was designed for in-patient groups: schizophrenics, drug addicts and then the terminally ill patients facing death. Frank Farrelly's approach (1974, 1987), Provocative Therapy, was developed for work with chronic schizophrenics to provoke an emotional response and to get the patient to laugh at his behavior through the therapists humorous verbal assault and antics.

Other individual therapists have developed humor models integrated into various psychotherapeutic models: Greenwald, Direct Decision Therapy (1973, 1987); Albert Ellis, Rational Emotive Therapy (1988); Salameh, Integrative Short-term Psychotherapy (1983, 1987); Madanes, Strategic Family Therapy (1987); Ventis, Behavior Therapy (1987); and Bloch, Group Therapy (1983, 1987). For an indepth review of these and others, I refer you to Kuhlman, T. L., 1984, *Humor and Psychotherapy* and Fry, W.F., Jr. & Salameh, W.A., 1987, *Handbook of Humor and Psychotherapy*.

In the therapeutic community approach to psychiatric treatment, there is an emphasis on a democratic and human orientation, the use of group psychotherapy and patient government, as well as other social concepts, i.e., patients assuming responsibility for their own behavior, for the welfare of others, and for group living. Within this setting, humor occurs and serves a social as well as psychological function.

The humor used by patients on one such ward in a VA hospital is described by Kaplan and Boyd (1965). The therapists felt that previous studies had ignored those functions of humor aimed at creating a feeling of intimacy and providing a means of winning social approval. Several needs of the patient groups were apparent: to adapt to the staff and others of the wider society; to restrain disruptive tendencies in the group; to alleviate personal anxiety; and to maintain a sense of solidarity.

Several themes in the expressed humor proved to be dominant. One was the "overdependence" allegedly fostered by the "comfortable" life of the VA hospital. The humor here served several functions; it reflected concern over possible maladaptation to the hospital; it assuaged the guilt associated with hospitalization; it reaffirmed the basic value of "wanting to get well;" and it served as an effective negative sanction against those who deviated from this value. The hospital was referred to as "Heroes Hotel," the "Neuropsychiatric Hilton," and the "Federal Womb."

Sex and obscenity was another common theme. Such joking was expected, since this was a male group; the infringement of a social taboo tends to make peer groups more cohesive and has "leveling" influence. It can be used as a "weapon" against the staff, but in such a way that it does not seriously disrupt the system. It also permits the patient group to identify with a normal group (the staff) by projecting on the staff the qualities the patients observe in themselves. One patient claimed he had a sex problem. "I've been screwed by the government for 15 years."

Humor about severe mental disorder was another theme. This humor served to allow dissociation from severe disturbance, and contributed toward cohesiveness and a social control function. The patients, however, ridiculed such behavior on other wards, but rarely their own group. Rather, when a disturbance did occur in their group, it was occasion for solicitude and giving of support.

Expressions of hostility through humor were also reported. When directed toward the staff, this kind of humor served as a morale booster among the patients. When expressed toward "civilians," it functioned to decrease the distance and the difference between them. The expression of hostile humor toward other patients helped to forestall deviant behavior and imposed a negative sanction. However, much of the humor directed toward other patients served to enhance the solidarity of the group by functioning as an initiation rite and to provide support, and as an expression of comradeship. They called the ward "Thorazine Hilton," and referred to projective tests as "those dirty pictures." When asked by a psychiatrist what he thought about calling doctors by their first names, one patient said, "John, I just don't feel right about calling you John." They controlled behavior of other patients by kidding them about that behavior — "telling tall tales," or being a "firebug." When new patients joined the group, older patients often introduced themselves as the ward psychiatrist or as Sigmund Freud. They played practical jokes on each other. Self-depreciating humor was used by patients either to deny the seriousness of their illness or to "accommodate" the staff.

However, it was felt that this self-ridicule permitted the person for the first time to take a detached view of himself and his problem; this recognition is the sine qua non of the therapeutic process. There seemed to be a relationship between the development of a sense of humor and "getting better."

The authors felt that the beneficial functions as well as the possible dysfunctional consequences of humor should be studied further as a consideration toward the facilitation of therapeutic progress.

Observing humor in group psychotherapy, Vargas (1961) saw it used in three ways: (1) to conceal some part of the personality which is considered distressing or undesirable, (2) to facilitate expression, and (3) to disguise yet express a feeling without overt commitment. He further elaborates on these. The patient may use humor to desensitize terms and concepts, to bring about a simple release of tension in the group, to express his judgment of events and conditions in the hospital, to facilitate the discussion of a frightening topic, or to provide the doorway by which he can enter into discussion of a serious problem.

The constructive use of humor in long-term insight group psychotherapy was identified by Bloch, et al, (1983) through their clinical experiences. Therapist-related uses are to model the humorous attitude, to show his "humanness," and as an avenue of interpretation. Patient-related uses are to give a sense of proportion; problems are seen in perspective, to overcome "earnestness;" a solemn, grave attitude to promote social skills and as a means of self-disclosure, which provides the relief or catharsis and can lead to further discussion. The humor can also play an important role in the life of the group as a whole, promoting group cohesion, giving insight into the group's dynamics, and as a strategy for reducing the unbearable tension which can arise.

These therapists also identified the potential "misuses of humor" in group therapy. The therapist-related misuses are:

— when it is used as defense against his own anxieties;

— to meet the therapist's need for expressing hostility; or

— to ingratiate himself with the group, or

— when there is confusion as to whether the therapist is serious or "just joking." Patients may use humor to block themselves from the therapeutic process by clowning, scapegoating one member of the group, or avoiding painful issues through self-mockery. The group as a whole can also abuse humor by avoidance of the serious work. The "fun" can be a temporary digression or respite from the hard work, but if continued can be maladaptive.

Humor in group psychotherapy also provides a means for controlling deviant behavior.

> In one therapeutic community where group psychotherapy included the total ward, newly admitted patients were simply included and introduced to the group. One day when a new patient was displaying very bizarre behavior, gesturing, posturing, etc., another patient finally leaned out and said to her, "Gladys, in this hospital you can be as crazy as you want, but, you can't act it! So, sit up!" At that point, the group laughed, but the patient sat up!

Warner (1984) discusses the therapeutic use of humor, within the milieu of a psychiatric setting, as a means of self-disclosure, utilizing such patient assignments as exploring favorite or offensive jokes and recall of humorous life events.

> Who is to say that mental illness is not a laughing matter, crazy talk is not funny and the whole subject should not be discussed openly? Maybe humor and openness should be acknowledged and used to benefit the client through mutual self-disclosures and shared laughter. "Laughing with" is not the same as "laughing at," and laughter is good for milieu as well as the soul.

As there is humor in this setting between patients, so there is humor among staff. As we indicated earlier, in such a stress-provoking setting, humor is common. A study conducted in 1954 analyzed the laughter in psychiatric staff conferences (Goodrich & Goodrich). Group laughter functioned as a mechanism to promote solidarity and provide a safety valve for divisive tensions. The major forms of humor were disparagement and incongruity. The commonest content of the laughter was at physicians and patients. There was a low percentage of laughter at sexual themes, but a heartiness of laughter at death. The social function of the laughter seemed to vary with the situation, e.g., a need for group tension release, uncertainty over a controversial issue, expression of a need for emotional support or to secure status, or a response to a violation of mores or of objective reality. The disparagement of patients by of mores or of objective reality. The disparagement of patients by the staff, which relieved their tensions and served the well-being of the group, placed a barrier between the patient and the personnel. Those listening to the case tended to lose sight of the disease process in the patient. This withdrawal from the patient's problems was deemed by the observers as an inappropriate response in view of therapeutic responsibilites.

Yet the relief from a difficult situation is as necessary for the staff as for the patient. In the milieu of a psychiatric hospital, Coser (1960) says, where the therapeutic process requires interactive competency, a staff member's every-day behavior has to be carefully controlled by himself and others. The self-consciousness and tension that arise under these conditions may seek release through humor.

In her study of the social functions of humor among the staff of a mental hospital during staff meetings, Coser found that humor among colleagues served to reduce the social distance — to relax the rigidity of the social structure without upsetting it. It served as a means of mutual reassurance, of asking for and giving support, of teaching and learning, of affirmation of common values in an area fraught with uncertainties.

Within the hierarchy of an organization like this mental hospital, she found the status structure was supported by downward humor. That is, those high in the hierarchy felt free to make the most witticisms, while those lowest on the authority structure made the fewest. Most of the witticisms were directed at some target: a patient, relatives, another staff member, or self. The least use of humor by those low on the staff did not mean they had less hostility and less need, but rather pointed out that role relationships within a situation control the behavior. The junior staff members were supposed to learn, to receive knowledge and to accept the intellectual superiority of the senior members. Too much humorous behavior would be interpreted as questioning the student-teacher relationship. The most frequent targets of the senior staff were the junior members, while the junior members directed their humor against patients, relatives, or themselves. Never was the humor within the meeting directed at an authority higher than the initiators.

Self-depreciating humor by a junior member, using himself as a target, pays respect to the system, but also decreases the social distance, because he permits authority an expression of its own aggression through laughter. The laughter of the authority figure grants the junior member's plea for needing to belong and strengthens the cohesion of the group.

Humor and laughter in the group may also dramatize a violation of a norm and, at the same time, reaffirm that norm. The humorist assumes the role of disguised moralist. The individual with a high staff position most often uses this role as a teaching device. The junior uses humor as a means of self-protection, a plea for sympathy. The laughter and humorous responses by the authority figure and the group combine criticism with support. This kind of humor informs the junior that it is not serious, that they can all laugh about it together, but at the same time points out the violation or blunder.

The junior member is in a paradoxical position. He has to assume the role of a student with his seniors, but to be a successful student, he must assume a professional, nonstudent role with his patients. The paradox may seek its solution in self-aggression against patients, but gets him the support and reassurance he needs, because it is an area around which consensus is easy. Coser says:

> The need for support is great indeed for those who have to deal with illness, especially in an area in which results are slow to be forthcoming and in which the therapist must constantly scrutinize and evaluate the techniques at his disposal (p. 91).

Humor is used as a device for lending support and for asking for support.

> The give and take of support through humor helps the participants to live up to role expectations and to overcome the contradictions and ambiguities inherent in the complex social structure, and therapy to contribute to its maintenance (p. 95).

The implications, then, for the education of the health professional through the use of humor are great. In an experiment conducted with first-year medical students comparing their future specialty choices with their attitudes toward death and appreciation of humor, O'Connell (1967) found potential psychiatrists did not have this same maturity and had higher concerns about their own deaths than any other specialty area. Potential surgeons had the lowest concerns about death! O'Connell suggests that potential psychiatrists may need education toward increased empathy and humor to make death concerns a professional asset. There is a need, he said, for "empathetic tutoring by exemplary figures to further develop empathy and humor (p. 441).

The relevance to education for all health professionals in all areas can be extrapolated from this base. In the next chapter we will attempt to describe this concept of humor in relation to the educational process of the health professional.

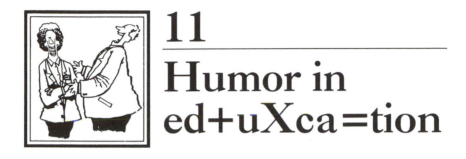

# 11
# Humor in
# ed+uXca=tion

*The Perception of the Comic is a tie of sympathy with other men, a*
*pledge of sanity. We must learn by laughter as well as by tears and*
*terror.*

Ralph Waldo Emerson

Another of the benefits of humor which has been identified by
many is that of facilitating or enhancing learning. "What is learned
with laughter is learned well" (Grotjahn, 1957, p. ix). Marshall
McLuhan (1967) said:

> Learning, the educational process, has long been associated
> only with the glum. We speak of the 'serious' student. Our
> time presents a unique opportunity for learning by means of
> humor — a perceptive or incisive joke can be more meaningful
> that platitudes lying between two covers (p. 10).

Carl Rogers (1969) stated that a sense of humor is one of the
essential qualities of that facilitator of learning, the teacher
(p. 108).

Extensive research by Avner Ziv, an Israeli psychologist, has demonstrated that humor does improve learning in school children and in adolescents and that humor is positively correlated with creativity (1976, 1979, 1980, 1983). A humorous approach stimulates divergent thinking, the creation of new ideas and new ways of looking at a situation. Laughter, he says, has a "liberating effect" on the flow of ideas. His studies have shown that the open, humorous teacher in the classroom is more effective in learning and in creating an atmosphere conducive to better academic work. Children love teachers who use humor in classes. Positive humor (not sarcasm or ridicule) that is relevant to what is being taught, improves learning.

Research by Zillman, Bryant (1983) demonstrated the positive effects of humor on learning with young children, even when not related to the material taught. With 5-6-year-olds, unrelated humor, when paced rapidly, enhanced their acquisition of information from educational television programs. However, the effect becomes weaker as the child's age increases. With adult, college-aged students, the humor must be "relevant" to the subject. Unrelated or irrelevant humor by the teacher detracts from the student-teacher rapport and has detrimental effects on the acquisition of information, whereas the involvement of relevant humor that is well integrated in the educational message may lead to superior retention of the educational information and is likely to make the learning experience more enjoyable and enhance the teacher-student rapport.

Ziv (1981, 1984) also demonstrated in a study with adolescents that humor may be a better predictor of leadership than IQ. The amateur humorists (those who are not professional comedians) have a more positive self-image and are often nominated by their peers for leadership roles.

And, of course, the physiological results of laughter in stimulating the production of the catacholamines and adrenaline in the brain (previously discussed), increases alertness and memory which enhances the learning process (Fry, 1986).

Despite the recognition of its importance, however, there has been little attempt by educators to make conscious, deliberate use of humor in the educational setting. The planned use of humor in the educational process of the health professional, as content in the curriculum and as an intervention tool to be used in health care, is still not a common occurrence in educational programs for the health professions.

The use of humor in the classroom by the teacher not only enhances learning and fosters the student-teacher relationship, but also provides the vehicle for developing the student's ability to relate in this warm and human way to others. The modeling of the use of humor by the instructor is also a first step in teaching the student in the helping professions how to utilize humor as a communication tool in intervening with patients in times of stress.

The socialization of students into the health professions begins the day they enters their first classroom. As we have discussed previously, they learn very quickly that humor is one way to cope with the "reality shocks" they encounter. The educational system has a responsibility to assist in this socialization process and it must assume responsibility for helping students learn to use this humor in an acceptable and constructive way.

There are four interrelated aspects to be considered in this area of education and humor:

1. Enhancing the learning process itself through humor.
2. Facilitating the process of socialization into the health profession through humor.
3. Teaching the concept of humor as a communication and intervention tool.
4. Modeling the use of humor as a vehicle for facilitating the other three.

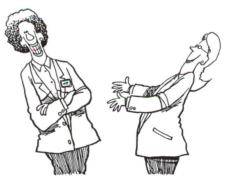

That humor must be a quality of any learning theory and certainly a necessary ingredient in learning about learning theories is the basis for Guy R. Lefrancois' book, *Psychological Theories and Human Learning:* Konger's Report (1972). The book is written as a report by an extraterrestrial being named Konger M-III 216, 784, 912, IVKX4 from the planet Koros. (Lefrancois "only collects the royalties.")

Although Lefrancois used humor very effectively in the teaching about learning theory, he did not relate the concept of humor per se to the framework of any learning theory.

It would seem, then, that rather than a relationship to one particular theory of learning, humor and laughter contribute to all those necessary principles of learning regardless of theory: enjoyment; interest; motivation; creativity; a relaxed, open, warm atmosphere; a positive student-teacher relationship; and reduced tension and anxiety.

Each of us subjectively can recall or relate some learning which we "will never forget" because it was presented in a humorous manner. The classic definition of menstruation as "the weeping of a disappointed uterus" not only produces a laugh, but conveys the physiology of the menstrual cycle in one short sentence to which the student can always relate.

Actually, if one were to relate humor to a particular learning theory, the humanistic approach to education would probably be the most appropriate. The humanistic perspective is looking toward man's capacity — what he can become rather than the normal, average, or adjusted individual. It is seeking to look at the here and now and the conscious self as opposed to the past orientation and the unconscious of the Freudians, and to look at what is going on inside the behavior rather than the observable behavior alone as the behaviorists do. Behavior from the humanistic stance is a result of our perceptions. What we perceive about ourselves constitutes our self-concept and affects how we behave. Similarly how we perceive others colors our interactions with them. Building a positive self-image; identifying that self-actualized man and how one produced him; exploring the meanings that lead to behavior, and finding meaning in one's life are the goals of the humanistic movement.

The implications of education are apparent, producing a fully functioning, self-actualized individual and mobilizing the potentials of every student. The teacher then becomes a facilitator of learning, not a director or information giver. He is a warm, caring person who is open, and provides the atmosphere in which the student can be involved in his own becoming and in developing a positive self-concept. The climate of the school from administrators to student is one of open communication, a respect for each other. Individualized instruction, self-pacing, self-discovery, self-management, learning from mistakes, fostering creativity, flexibility, and encouraging the development of personal meaning in learning are all techniques of the humanistic approach to education.

Abraham Maslow (1970), who pioneered the humanistic movement, has defined self-actualized man as having a philosophical, unhostile sense of humor; the ability not only to poke fun at himself, but of having a sense of humor which reminds others of their "humanness." He defines humor and laughter as "education in a palatable form" (p. 169-170).

Being real and genuine is one of the qualities or attitudes of a teacher who facilitates learning, and having a sense of humor is an aspect of being genuine, says Carl Rogers. He quotes a student's reaction: "Your sense of humor in the class was cheering; we all felt relaxed because you showed us your human self, not a mechanical image" (1969, p. 108).

Kenneth Eble in his book, "The Perfect Education" (1966), says laughter creates the very air in which learning thrives. He feels laughter must begin in the home and continue throughout education. Laughter frees up and opens pathways to creativity and discovery. He beseeches parents to shake off the habit of excessive worry and pushing.

> More positively, they must laugh greatly. For children, solemnity is like a whole pane of glass in an abandoned building. Solemnity invites shattering . . . .
>
> But why laughter? Because laughter is giving and recognizing. It forces a physical giving that releases for a moment the very self. And if we did not recognize some rugged corner of ourselves, some flawed reality, we would not laugh. Such giving is necessary to prepare the self to learn . . . . Parents can hardly do better than respond to their children's sense of absurdity, to let physical ticklings grow into wit, to let wit grow into a sense of the world as it is and as it should be (p. 204).

He advises parents to consider laughter even before love because laughter keeps love from smothering, and if we laugh, we are bound to love. He says ". . . laughter makes parenthood bearable . . . ." If laughter is not linked with learning at home, the connection is not likely to be made in school.

> Surely the thing that drives hundreds of bright, laughing college students out of the colleges of education is the solemnity of their utterances as well as their behavior (p. 15).

Education [should] keep us alive and hopeful . . . and lead us
to laugh in the face of heaven or hell. For serious as our
strivings are, they should never be so serious that we cannot
lean back and laugh at the absurdity of our being and doing.
Education should teach us to play the wise fool rather than
turn us into the solemn ass (p. 214).

The concepts inherent in the humanistic approach to education
are ones that have been closely related to the concept of humor.
The perception of ourselves and how others perceive us, the
loving, caring, warm atmosphere, and the concepts of creativity
and change — are evidenced in both.

The use of humor is a mechanism which does not destroy one's
self-image, but provides a way to criticize, show mistakes, and
express values, yet save face for the individual and imply a loving
relationship in doing so. It's all right. You made a mistake, just
something to laugh about, to learn from. No harm done. You are not
a terrible person, just human. Coser (1960), in the study of humor
between colleagues (discussed in the previous chapter), describes
this use of humor as a teaching device which not only helps to
resolve the paradoxical role of the student, who, to be a good
student must also be a professional, but also serves as an informal
process of socialization into the profession.

The teacher relating humorous experiences of his own which
often show "boo-boos" and mistakes he has made, helps the
student, who usually has unrealistic expectations of his own
performance, to relax and accept the learning process.

The students' imitations and mimickings of instructors and
hospital staff (a common practice in health professions), seen not
only in private but at school parties where the subjects of the humor
are present, demonstrate the relationship in reverse; that is, the
students are able to express their own hostility, to criticize and
relieve their anxiety and tension, yet show affection and warmth.
Many of the "scenes" in the acting reveal the areas around which
the most anxiety for the student has taken place. (A clue for the
educator to heed in future teaching!) These humorous plays and
skits also are part of the socialization process: "We're one of you
now. We can laugh about it with you!" The student who can
initiate humor comfortably with faculty gives evidence of an
interpersonal skill that will be reflected in his ability to relate to

other people.

The concepts of creativity and change are closely related to each other as well as to humor and learning. Creativity implies the ability to change and produce change. To be a change agent implies the ability to be creative.

> We are . . . faced with an entirely new situation in education where the goal of education, if we are to survive, is the facilitation of change and learning. The only man who is educated is the man who has learned how to learn . . . how to adapt to change . . . realized that no knowledge is secure, that only the process of seeking knowledge gives a basis for security (Rogers, 1969, p. 104).

The humorous release, says Mindess, is:

> . . . change of venue . . . the sober citizen having gotten the point of a jest, merely exchanges his ordinary outlook for a broader, subtler, or more novel one. Breaking loose from one set, we settle for another . . . the delight is in the process, in the experience of change (1971, p. 142).

To cultivate our sense of humor requires that we learn to thrive on change, Mindess adds.

The aspect of creativity in both learning and humor is obvious. The very act of producing humor or comedy is creativity in itself. Koestler (1964) and Fry (1963) both speak of humor as an act of creation which requires the ability to abstract and conceptualize. Enjoyment of humor, to get the point of a joke, requires the same ability. The procedure of humor is the procedure for creativity,

> . . . for in its construction as well as its content, the ludicrous continually provides us with new compositions formed out of old raw materials . . . as a body of activity our indulgence in humor facilitates our creative possibilities, for it lubricates the unconventional, imaginative problem-solving functions of our being (Mindess, 1971, p. 153-154).

It "paves the way for originality on a wider scale" and "has the power to unlock all our other creative potentials," Mindess concludes.

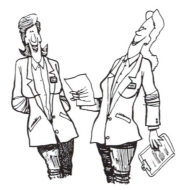

We have suggested that, through the use of humor, the educational process begins the socialization of the student into the "reality shocks" he faces. In our teaching in those areas, which create the social conflicts both student and patient face, a bit of humor facilitates an understanding and may even lead to a discussion of these conflicts.

For example, a comment used by an instructor in a lecture to beginning nursing students: "On Monday we will have a discussion of vomiting, including a practical demonstration of the technique," not only produces a laugh, but in effect says, "I know vomiting isn't a pleasant subject or one which you have been in the habit of dealing with, so let's laugh a little about it." There could follow, then, a discussion of the student's reaction, the patient's reaction, and the responsibilities of a professional in managing this unpleasant situation.

Similarly, in a class on the procedure of giving of an enema, one instructor began her discussion of the psychosocial implications with, "How would you approach a patient to whom you are giving an enema? Would you say, 'Ha! Ha! Look what I've got for you!'" The students' laughter is acknowledgment of their anxiety in facing the embarrassment and conflict of this situation. Acceptance of humor as one way of coping can be discussed as well as recognizing that the patient may also joke in the situation, and that the student can feel comfortable in responding. Serious discussion of all the implications involved in this procedure as well as others can ensue.

One of the contentions of many educators is that education is a "serious" business, and that scientific and medical subjects, particularly, do not lend themselves to humor. However, this has been refuted by many authors. Even "dull," somber, scientific subjects can be lightened by humor. It is a fallacy that there are "proper" subjects for jokes, while others are too sacred to talk about. It is the time and place which are the decisive factors, not the subject.

A textbook on the use of computers in data processing in education in discussing the use of base 10 in mathematics says:

> There is nothing particularly sacred about a base of 10. Probably the only reason it was originally developed and is now in widespread use is that man happens to have 10 fingers. Other systems have been created. For example, the Babylonians had a base of 60 (of course, they also did their writing on mud pies); the Mayas of Yucatan used a base of 20 (warm climate and groups of barefooted mathematicians?); and a base of five is still used by natives in New Hebrides (one hand is wrapped around a spear and is thus not available for counting?) (Sanders, 1973, p. 147).

In the medical field, not all situations or human diseases lend themselves to humor, but even there a relatively somber, scientific discussion as to why the sphincter ani must be preserved when performing surgery in that area was described by Bornemeier in an amusing style:

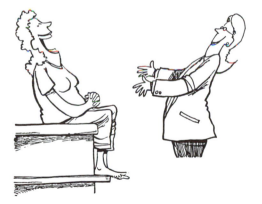

> They say man has succeeded where the animal fails because of the clever use of his hands, yet when compared to the hands, the sphincter ani is far superior. If you place into your cupped hands a mixture of fluid, solid and gas and then through an opening at the bottom, try to let only the gas escape, you will fail. Yet the sphincter ani can do it. The sphincter apparently

can differentiate between solid, fluid and gas. It apparently can tell whether its owner is alone or with someone, whether standing up or sitting down, whether its owner has his pants on or off. No other muscle in the body is such a protector of the dignity of man, yet so ready to come to his relief. A muscle like this is worth protecting (1960, p. 45-52).

Robert Baker (1967), who believes that science and humor are not mutually contradictory, put together a collection of scientific humor in a book entitled, *A Stress Analysis of a Strapless Evening Gown and Other Essays for a Scientific Age*. The essays include such intriguing titles as "The Lab Coat as Status Symbol" by F. E. Warburton; "Parkinson's Laws in Medical Research" by C. Northcote Parkinson; "Saga of a New Hormone" by Norman Applezweig; and "Body Ritual Among the Nacirema" by Horace Miner. Baker says:

> . . . both scientists and satirists [are] dedicated to the proposition that neither science nor man can hope to survive the rigors of our age without a sense of humor (p. ix).

Another collection of humorous essays by Baker (1963) is called *Psychology in the Wry*. It was assembled, he says, because too many professional psychologists and their students have not only forgotten how to laugh, but also believe it is unscientific to do so. The contributors represent many branches of psychology, and have created this new branch, a science of satire, in defense of psychology's mental health. One article entitled, "Sidesteps Toward a Nonspecial Theory" by Edgar F. Borgatta, presents some theories Freud overlooked: deumbilification, mammary envy, digital gratification, and the no-person group.

Humorous journals and magazines have surfaced. *The Journal of Polymorphous Perversity* publishes humorous and satirical works in the field of psychology, psychiatry and other allied disciplines. *The Journal of Irreproducible Results* lampoons scientific research.

A series of textbooks written in a humorous manner, whose purpose is to enhance the learning, have been developed by Med-Master, Inc., publishers. They include: *Clinical Anatomy and Physiology for the Frustrated Health Professional* (Stewart, 1986); *Psychiatry Made Ridiculously Simple* (Good & Nelson, 1984); and *The*

*4-Minute Neurologic Exam* (Goldberg, 1984).

When teaching in a scientific, somber, or delicate area such as health or disease, one must always balance between achievement of a goal and a need for tact in the use of the humor to avoid misunderstandings and offending sensibilities. Yet, as Reese (1967) summed up the case for humor in medicine:

> I would never suggest that the physician writer not take his medicine seriously. I do hope, however, he will occasionally laugh at himself, amuse his readers when it helps to get and hold their attention, warm up his facts before he serves them, and use humor whenever it adds a touch of humanity (p. 13).

In this chapter, we have expressed a belief that humor does have a valuable place in education. How the educator can learn to model it and teach the use of humor as a tool in communication, and how humor can be used in patient education, will be discussed in Section III, "Cultivating the Use of Humor."

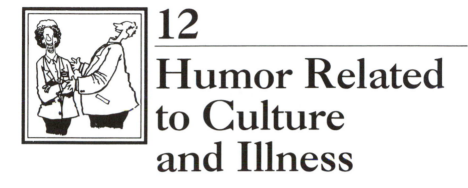

# 12
# Humor Related to Culture and Illness

One of the variables always to be considered in planning health care is the cultural background of the patient and family. Each culture has practices and beliefs which influence the reaction to illness and to health care. Health personnel must be as sensitive to the cultural needs of people as they are to the physical, psychological, and social needs. "Today, more than ever before, there is a need to understand people from different cultures and to use this knowledge in the helping process" (Leininger, 1970, p. 45).

> Cultural differences are often the basis for poor communication, interpersonal tensions, and hesitation in working effectively with others. Cultural similarities make us appreciate humanness, common human bonds, and behavior features which point to human universality (Ibid, p. vii).

The humor within cultures, and the similarities and differences, then, must also be a factor to be considered in the planned use of humor in interactions with patients and their families. Is there a difference in the kind of humor which emanates from a particular culture or ethnic group? Does culture or ethnicity make a difference in the kind of humor which is appreciated? Are there similarities or are there universal topics for humor? Is there a relationship between a specific culture and its use of humor in times of stress-like illness? If so, what is it? Would the culture of the patient make a difference in the health professional's use of humor if the professional were a nonmember of the culture?

Definitive answers to these questions, as with most others in this area of humor, are not available. There are the same varied opinions and generalizations. Specific studies regarding humor and cultural or ethnic groups are rare, and comprehensive studies regarding cultural groups and their use of humor in relation to health and illness, are apparently nonexistent.

"Extensive analyses of the many characteristics of humor in individual cultures are rare, and cross-cultural studies of humor simply do not exist" (Apte, 1984, p. 9). Yet we know that smiling and laughter transcend cultures and that humor is a molding force in all societies. The popular humor of a people often expresses their concerns, conflicts and aspirations. We can hypothesize that there will be differences, but that there will also be similarities since laughter is a universal human behavior (Levine, 1968, Grotjahn, 1957).

This dichotomy of humor is illustrated by the Greenland Eskimos who resolve their quarrels by duels of laughter. Each recites humorous insults and obscene jokes ridiculing his opponent. The one who gets the most laughs from the audience wins. The other, humiliated, often goes into exile.

Some types of humor, however, seem to transcend cultures. Charlie Chaplin, during a visit to a primitive tribe in East Africa, was expected to respond in kind after their dance performance for him. He chose to dance for them his pantomine of a bullfight. The natives roared with laughter. He then went one step farther, and performed a bedroom farce of a woman caught by her husband in bed with her lover. This act also was understood and resulted in hilarity.

Nearly every society has developed some form of institutional-ized humor as a method of social release and regulation. Radcliffe-Brown in 1940 first described the "joking relationship" from his study of primitive tribes in Africa. This social relationship has been found to be widespread in all societies. He defined the term as "a relation between two persons in which one is by custom permitted, and in some instances required, to tease or make fun of the other, who in turn is required to take no offense" (1952, p. 90). There are two varieties. In the symmetrical, both participants can tease and make fun of each other. In the asymmetrical, one teases the other who either can accept it good-humoredly without retaliating or only teases back a little. In some instances, the joking and teasing are only verbal; in others there is horse-play, and still others include elements of obscenity. The joking relationship is a peculiar combination of friendliness and antagonism. It is one of "permitted disrespect." This is important, Levine (1961) says, because the "maintenance of a social order depends upon the appropriate kind and degree of respect being shown towards certain persons, things and ideas or symbols" (p. 91).

This teasing and joking relationship performs a vital function in defining and maintaining kinship relationships. It also provides the culture with external controls for the sexual and aggressive urges that would violate the rules of that culture if expressed directly. In many of our American Indian tribes, the ritual clown is a highly respected individual who, in his antics as part of the ceremonies of the tribe, is permitted to violate every social taboo. Such a relationship provides a vicarious release for the audience.

We identify various types of jokes by their ethnic or national character. We speak of Irish jokes, Jewish jokes, Scottish jokes, German jokes, English jokes, etc. These jokes may reveal the personality or character traits, the stereotypes or the conflicts of that particular group. These may be reflected in the style of humor or the content. Although the functions of humor are universal, there are differences in national style (Ziv, 1988). The greatest differences among cultures are found in the content and situations of humor and depends on their cultural histories, he says. Jokes about drinking are found in Irish humor, but are practically non-existent in Israeli humor. Sexual, aggressive humor predominates in American humor, but not in less aggressive nations like Japan or Belgium. French humor is often sexual, British humor more intellectual. Tall tales and exaggerations are typical of "pioneer" nations such as the United States, Australia and Israel, but rare in "older" nations (p. xi).

Mikes (1971) feels that people all over the world laugh at the same things, but there are some jokes which reflect the national character. A crook or cheat is always portrayed as fair in an English joke, whereas he is clever in a Jewish joke. The victim is seen as stupid in the German version of the joke. Understatement is the style of the British; overstatement, exaggeration, and leg-pulling characterize the style of the American. The love of self-mockery and self-criticism is shared by both English and Jews.

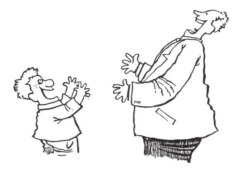

The Jews needed jokes, Mikes contends. It was the only way they could survive through thousands of years of persecution, the only way to save their self-respect and to laugh at their tormentors. There are many jokes about anti-Semitism and superior Jewish cleverness. This is a preventative mechanism that wards off anticipated attack, has pride as well as humility, and pleads for love. It creates for the Jews a bond and a solidarity. Tell a Jewish joke to an anti-Semite, Mikes contends, and if he laughs he will be less anti-Semitic. A reflection of the change in their social situation, Jewish humor, says Mikes, has been lost in transit to Israel. Jews in Israel are no longer oppressed. Humor still survives, but the difference is seen in this joke:

> An Israeli couple is touring Europe with their 11-year-old child. He asks in Italy, Germany, Holland, Sweden, "Are these people Jews?" He is told each time, "No, they are Christians." The boy, with sympathy, finally says, "Poor Christians. It must be awful for them to be scattered like that all over the world" (p. 115).

Ziv (1988) says "Israeli" humor developed from the rich tradition of Jewish humor, but the "extreme seriousness" of the pioneers in building a new homeland and a "new Jew" did not leave much place for self-disparagement (p. 122). Aggressive humor and social humor have taken the place of "loving satire" and self-disparagement.

Humor has served similar functions for other minority cultures. Many comedians and analysts of comedy claim that humor has done more to change the status of minority groups and reduce racial prejudice than any other factor. Black comedians feel wit and humor are better weapons and a greater force than anger in easing racial tension.

Investigation of humor in relation to the issue of racial prejudice in minority cultures has been the focus of several studies and writings over the years. Myrdal (1944), in the context of race relations, described a number of social functions provided by intergroup humor: as an escape route, as compensation to the sufferer, as absolution provided in the form of an understanding laugh, and as indirect approval for that which cannot be explicitly acknowledged (pp. 38-39).

In the history of racial conflict humor has played a definite role (Burma, 1946). It lends itself well to use as a conflict device because of its boundless limits in subject matter, and because its nature is such that it often contains more or less well-concealed malice. Burma discusses particularly "Negro-White" humor which makes one or the other the butt of the humor. The notion of Negroes lampooning whites may come as a surprise. Yet for many decades Negroes were usually in a position in which their conflict and defense techniques had to be covert. This favored the growth of a more subtle type of humor as a weapon of both offense and defense.

Prejudice, both racial and cultural, provides a fertile field for the folklorist. Folktales created by minority groups toward whom prejudice is shown function through sarcasm, humor, or parody to preserve the ego identity of the minority group. This type of humor conserves mental health through sublimation, allowing release of the suppressed anger via protest humor (Simmons, 1963).

These tales utilize several techniques. One may state that personal salvation is to be found only within the minority group and that anyone who adopts the customs of the majority group is lost. Another tale may involve trickster motifs by which a member of the group successfully counters an insult by the majority group. Another may parody an alleged stereotype or follow a majority group logic to an unexpected conclusion. A fifth may denigrate the majority group.

In summary, humor functions in intergroup conflict as a mechanism for expressing aggression toward an out-group. This is done through the use of sarcasm and ridicule; enhancing the morale of the in-group, and undermining the morale of those against whom the humor is directed. In addition, humor may serve as a means of accommodation, as the Negro slave appeased his white master through self-ridicule and self-debasement.

# A STUDY OF THREE CULTURES

If comprehensive studies and analyses of humor in specific cultures are rare, the use of humor in times of illness in specific cultures is even more rare. To provide some beginning base for consideration of the variable of cultures in using humor as a tool in communication, a concentration on a small number of cultures was thought to be more fruitful. The problem was approached by looking first for specific studies of humor in that culture, and then reviewing the literature on health and illness in that culture, in an attempt to find any references to the use of humor, or any correlations between the two. As a third step, a small study was conducted (in 1975) to attempt to collect some original data.

Since national humor (Irish, Scottish, French, English, German, and the like) has been more or less accepted and incorporated into the Anglo-Saxon melting pot of our western culture, it was felt that reviewing specific minority cultures within our American society would be more meaningful. Consequently, three cultures were chosen: Black-American, Spanish-American, and Southwest Indian. Each would have, as a similar component, the use of humor as a minority group.

The Southwest Indian was chosen since there are differences recognized by anthropologists and linguists between various Indian groups. In the Southwest Indian group, the literature relates more specifically to the Navajo.

Spanish-American and Black-American are compromise terms and are used in a broad sense to define those two groups. There are many distinctions made and many individual preferences expressed.

Leininger makes a distinction between Spanish-Americans, who are descendents of the Spanish colonists, the Mexican-Americans who migrated from Mexico, and the Mexicans. Each have their own heritage and differences, yet there are similarities in belief, and all are Spanish-speaking. Nava separates the Mexican-American from other Spanish-surnamed, stating that they represent several races and different cultures. Most are mestizos, part Spanish and part Indian, but some are pure Indian and some pure Spanish. The younger generation today prefer to be called Chicano, reflecting the more aggressive stance, rejecting assimilation into the Anglo culture, and demanding respect for their bicultural identity. Individuals differ widely in their preferences. Some prefer Spanish-American, others Mexican-American or Hispano, Latino or Chicano. Some reject the term Chicano because of its militant connotation. Others prefer either the Spanish or Mexican term, reflecting whether they feel their heritage is Spanish or Mexican.

Similarly, in the Black-American group, there are variations. Some groups prefer Afro-American rather than Black, reflecting their African heritage. Negro is still used in many studies as an anthropological term, even though Black has become a widely preferred term. "Black" has been adopted by the new generation in their militant movement to gain equality and respect, i.e., "Black is beautiful." Here again, there are individual preferences. One very indignant young lady said, "I am Negro! See that skin It's not black! And, I don't dress, think, or act like the 'Blacks." However, terms like colored are universally resented.

Because of the association of most of these terms with minority, which can perpetuate the feelings of inferiority and discrimination, the Western Council on Higher Education for Nursing suggested that the term ethnic groups of color be used to begin to create a change in attitude. In the exploratory study conducted by this author, the terms Black-American, Spanish-American, and Indian-American were established after preliminary discussions with various groups and individuals. In every pre- and post-interview, reactions to these terms were solicited. Often a spontaneous reaction occurred prior to the discussion. One individual also reacted to the term Anglo as discriminatory!

The exploratory study was designed to collect humorous incidents in health settings when the patient was from one of these three cultures. The purpose was to provide some beginning data to answer the question of whether the culture of the patient makes a difference in the use of humor by the patient or health professional.

Three health agencies agreed to participate in the study: a large general hospital in the inner city area, a public health agency in a predominantly black residential district, and a neighborhood health center in a predominantly Spanish-American community. Despite the enthusiasm of the 60 health professionals who agreed to collect data, only 15 actual incidents were reported. The study suffered from the same problems of investigation described in the first chapter. Information gathered in pre- and post-interviews provided many more recollections of incidents which had occurred in the past, as well as personal opinions and thoughts regarding the differences and similarities.

## Southwest Indian

Of the three groups, the Indian culture is the only one in which an anthropological study of humor had been conducted. Extensive studies of the Navajo Indian culture were done in the 1940s (Kluckhohn & Leighton, 1946; Leighton & Leighton, 1944; Thompson, 1946).

> A popular fallacy has long existed that the American Indian is a stolid, unemotional individual incapable of expression or appreciation of humor or wit. Nothing is farther from the truth. Examples taken from the Navaho show that, in his own social sphere, the Indian can and does scintillate in conversation and in action in a manner comparable to that of peoples of European cultures. His humor runs the gamut of puns, practical jokes, and obscenities. In addition, he is an excellent mimic and pantomimist with a superb sense of timing and climax (Hill, 1943, p. 7).

Others describe the Navajo's keen sense of humor as having a whimsical quality that is seldom cruel. Wit and repartee are highly valued in conversation. Between relatives, a patterned type of teasing occurs. All types of humor are indulged in and reacted to by all classes and ages of persons. There is less difference due to age, sex, and social position than in white society. A respected older man often acts the buffoon. However, the Navajo does not like to be laughed at, and he wants to be well regarded, particularly by his white friends.

The importance of laughter as a social communication device can be illustrated by the practice of providing a festive meal for the family, prepared by the person who elicits a baby's first laugh. It is marked as a milestone and occasion in the baby's life.

The clown is a very important institution in the Navajo culture and is a vital part of the religious rituals (Reichard, 1950). Religion and illness are very closely related and medicine or treatment is administered with much ceremony by the clowns who are impersonating the gods. The ritualistic process ejects the evil and the good is absorbed by the patient. A person subjected to a ceremony thus possesses a great many powers to keep him safe. Sandpainting is one such ceremony in which the sand absorbs the evil and the patient absorbs the good of the supernaturals represented by the sand.

The study conducted by Kluckhohn and Leighton (1946) was an analysis of the Indian service program. The shortcomings of the program were a result of the failure to understand the cultural patterns of the Navajo. The health program particularly was adversely affected by not taking into consideration the beliefs around illness and disease.

Among the beliefs is the idea that the individual is a unit; therefore, parts of the body should not be treated separately. The Navajo "Singers" or medicine men, who cured with rituals, treated patients accordingly, whereas white doctors were apt to treat specific illnesses.

That nature is more powerful than man is a theme which pervades the whole culture, and the supernatural fears and beliefs extend to illness and disease. There is a belief that by witchcraft evil men and women can produce the illness or death of those whom they hate. Since there is no belief in immortality, death and everything connected with it are abhorred by the Navajo. There is a fear of ghosts, the dead who may return to plague the living. Therefore, a disease or injury is not caused by some physiological process, but rather by a violation of one of the taboos or beliefs, by a ghost or by witchcraft. The treatment then is to appease the supernaturals. The aim of the curing ceremonials is to restore the patient to a normal condition in his supernatural relationships. The Navajo highly values health and strength, and fears disease and injury. However, he rarely shares his beliefs with the white man because they are sacred and not to be readily shared with just anyone.

It is a great disappointment to the Indian people that the granite-faced grunting redskin stereotype still has been perpetuated, says Vine Deloria, a Sioux (1964). Indians have found a humorous side to nearly every problem, he says, and use teasing as a method of controlling social situations. Today, humor occupies a prominent place in national Indian affairs. Tribes are brought together by sharing humor of the past. "Columbus" jokes gain great sympathy, as well as jokes about the Bureau of Indian Affairs and General Custer. Tribes enjoy teasing each other. They agree that humor is the cement that holds the Indian movement together.

Vine Deloria speaks for the New Indian: the one who is no longer fighting for physical survival, but for ideological survival. The new generation of university-educated Indians has given voice to a human morality and tribal philosophy of life that weds the ancient with the modern. These young educated Indians are going back to be tribal leaders, to teach, to practice medicine and nursing, and to build educational facilities and health care services for their people.

There is a change in the medical behavior of the Navajo today (Steiner, 1968). Western medicine is accepted. However, the Navajo still believes strongly in his own religion, and rituals and medicine are still closely intertwined. The "Singer" and "Hand Trembler" are still very much a part of health care. When this does not work, scientific medicine is another means of treatment. There is a change also in that the Singer or Hand Trembler may suggest the patient go to the clinic or hospital. It must be recognized that religious rituals have a strong therapeutic effect and there is great support gained by the presence of all the family and friends who gather to help. The health professional needs to understand and accept this mixture (Adair, Denschle, 1970).

In this author's small study, five humorous incidents involving the Indian were reported. Three of these reflected the minority feelings and the teasing of the white man.

> When the Indian patient was asked about his name "Limpy," he proceeded to tell the story of his great-grandfather who fought at the Little Big Horn massacre and was given the name Limpy by his ancestors when he wounded a white man, causing him to limp!

> Another Indian patient with a scar on his back made jokes about "being knifed in the back."

> The third incident occurred between a Crow Indian nurse's aide and a white patient. The aide had entered the room with another aide, who was Filipino. The patient teasingly asked if there were any Americans around. The Indian aide responded with, "What do you mean? I'm the first American!"

> In the fourth incident, the patient was a Kickapoo Indian who upon being told that the tumor she had was not malignant, sighed with relief and said, "I thought I had swallowed a snake." The nurse reacted with surprise rather than laughter and the patient had to say, "That's a joke!"

Although the nurse did not pursue this "joke," we might speculate on its significance to the culture. According to the Indian culture, snakes are realistically feared, but are to be avoided rather than killed. It is a taboo to kill many creatures. Eating them is definitely a taboo. The patient may have been making a joke about the superstitious belief that violation of a taboo had caused her illness. However, the nurse did not understand this, and therefore did not "get the joke."

The fifth incident involved a Kickapoo Indian child playing hide and seek with the school nurse each time the child was to receive her medication. The incident appeared to be typical child's play.

These examples, as small as they are, reflect the admixture of old culture and new.

## Spanish-American Culture

Anthropological studies and literature on the use of humor in the Spanish-American culture are nonexistent. More literature is available describing the relationship of the culture to health and illness. References to joking and teasing as a way to indoctrinate the young into the culture, in family relationships, and in peer relationships, are alluded to indirectly in a study by Madsen (1964). Much kidding and joking among males occurs as a way to show respect for courage, for "machismo," and for being a "true man," that is, to drink more, to defend himself better, and to be more virile than any other man. The male is jokingly compared to a rooster. The woman, on the other hand, is to be submissive, weak, and "pure." A loose woman is often the object of jest and ridicule. One might expect that a woman in this culture rarely teases or jokes with the man.

Humor also serves as a leveling mechanism. Achievements, better position, and more wealth create envy, considered a destructive emotion. Therefore, one must not flaunt his success, rather he should play down his achievements, or others will do so through teasing.

Pedro, who came into the Cantina dressed in a new suit, was teased about "running for mayor." "Pedro has come into money. The drinks are on him" (Ibid, p. 23).

Joking is also used as a way to solidify the cohesiveness of the culture, ridiculing Anglo behavior, implying it is good to be Mexican.

The written humor or comedy has generally come out of Mexico, South America, or Cuba. Comic books are read extensively by the masses in Mexico, and are used as a means of social commentary and political satire. A poster of cartoons in Spanish, Chistes, published by the Spanish Poster Service of Homestead, Florida, reflects both the American culture and the Spanish. One cartoon shows a family portrait in color in which all the family is white with one fellow dressed in black with long black hair, mustache and beard. The caption is Oveja Negra (the Black Sheep). It conveys several messages. One is the incongruity of applying the term "black sheep" to humans in a family portrait. But the changing values and attitudes are also conveyed: the move from being "white" and fair in color, which has been an admired characteristic in Spanish and Latin American countries to the new generation's respect for being dark-skinned. The new Chicano often calls himself Brown.

The cultural beliefs of the Spanish-American around health and illness have been well described. These beliefs are in many ways similar to those of the Navajo. Religion, rituals, folk medicine and curing, and the belief that man has only limited control over nature are similarities that greatly affect the response to illness and health care.

The Spanish-American views himself as a passive victim of malevolent forces in his environment. God gives health and also sends illness. The illness may be viewed as a punishment from God or as a cross to bear. One patient believed he was paralyzed by polio because he kicked at his mother. Other illnesses may be caused by witchcraft or by careless or malicious behavior of others. Therefore, one is not to be blamed for being ill because of a personal lack of care or neglect.

*Mal ojo* or evil eye is an illness (usually in children) that is caused by someone admiring the child to an excessive degree. The prevention or cure is to have that person touch the admired or afflicted one. Empacho is a condition in which contaminated food is given to an individual because of maliciousness, while mal de susto (illness of fright) is caused by some emotional and frightening experience. Maleficio (or witchcraft) can be caused by malicious friends or witches. Some witches produce pain by forcing an evil wind (mal aire) to enter a victim's body. Prayers, ritual acts, folk medicine, and folk practitioners are used in the treatment of these illnesses. The curandero, medico, sobador, or albolario are used to diagnose as well as treat.

There is little emphasis on illness in the future; rather, illness is viewed as being in the present. Therefore, preventative practices, like immunizations, are not viewed with the same concern as the health professional views them. Keeping the mind and body in balance in order to be healthy, however, is important. The balances of "hot" and "cold" in relation to the body, to foods, and to interpersonal relationships are well defined.

The family is also an important consideration in making decisions and in giving support during times of illness. The patient does not deal with illness alone. The Spanish-American, therefore, expects that the curer or health professional will be warm and friendly and interested in all aspects of his life, as the curandero and his family are. The therapist must not be too impersonal and clinical. And, above all, he must not laugh at or ridicule the patient's beliefs. As with the Navajos, changes in medical beliefs and scientific medical practice have been accepted, but there is a mixture of both that must be recognized by the professional.

Some of these beliefs and attitudes are reflected in the humorous incidents reported and the opinions expressed by the health personnel in the study. One of the Mexican-American nurses felt that one must be careful in using humor with the Spanish-American because it may be taken seriously, especially if it indicates any kind of blame. Illness is often regarded as a form of punishment. Joking, she found, was used mainly as a denial of illness and of its seriousness. But once accepted, the laughter often turns to tears. This is the reason many patients do not come to the clinic until very seriously ill. She gave several examples:

> A young adolescent girl with a lump in her breast joked about having only one breast and what her boyfriend would do.

> A male patient with a bleeding ulcer joked about getting drunk and eating too much chili; if the nurse would come and cook for him, he would be fine.

Another cardiac patient who had been put on a regimen of restricted activity and diet following surgery, was brought in from a bar where he had collapsed. He joked about having to drink to keep up his "machismo," and teased the nurse about coming home to take care of him.

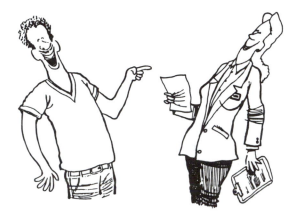

The husband of a patient who had cancer of the cervix had initially refused to let his wife go to the hospital, wanting more children, afraid his wife was not "going to be a woman." He joked with the nurse in a flirtatious way about being a woman. The nurse related that she had had a hysterectomy and asked if she "was less than a woman, now."

Several other examples from the study have to do with male manliness and male-female relationships:

A 14-year-old adolescent male was given a pre-football physical examination by the nurse practitioner. When she asked him to lower his shorts so that she could check for a hernia, he hesitated, and then asked if the other boys had allowed her to do this. Finally he said, "Well, it's okay but I'm not going to look!"

Another older Spanish-American male patient tease the male aide who was removing his cast about not getting too close to certain parts of his body.

Another Spanish-American male patient who was recovering from knee-cartilage surgery was asked by the Spanish-American nurse's aide how he was doing. He laughed and said, "Not so good, I can't get my leg up to make love to my wife."

In pre- and post-interviews with the staff from the Spanish-American Clinic and other Spanish-American health personnel, the question was asked whether they felt there was a difference in the humor used by the culture if the professional was a nonmember of the culture. The responses varied from 'no difference' to 'yes.'

One professional, a white, said she had heard the same Polack joke in South America that she heard in Wisconsin, except that the local minority group in that country had been substituted for Polack: "Where would you hide money from a Polack? Under a cake of soap."

The Mexican-American nurse, on the other hand, felt there was a difference if the professional was a nonmember, particularly in male-female interaction. The Spanish-American male may joke with her, but such behavior from an Anglo may be misinterpreted and taken seriously. She gave an example:

> A young Anglo laboratory technician was very solicitous of a young Spanish-American male who had been brought in with an overdose of drugs, and teased him as he was recovering. The patient became very upset when she subsequently rejected his request to take her out.

In a discussion of cultural beliefs, the head nurse, who was white, said, "You know, I may have innocently put the *mal ojo* on babies and children, because I didn't know." One of the Chicano staff laughed and said, "Oh, we know how stupid Anglos are, so it doesn't bother us."

The implications from this discussion are that there must be trust and respect before humor will be understood and acceptable. Even a Spanish professional must know the patient well. In the case of a nonmember this relationship is even more crucial.

## Black-American Culture

In reviewing the literature of the Black-American culture, humor has been integrated into all the other issues surrounding the history of the Black man in this country, and reflects the changes which have occurred. The original anthropological studies describing the joking relationship were observed in African tribes. Africa is the origin of the Black-Americans of today. However, the humor patterns of that culture could hardly be transposed to the new culture and circumstances in which the black slave found himself on these shores, since the situation and the relationships determine a joke culture. Perhaps the one aspect that has remained is the ability to laugh at harsh reality and tragedy. Anthropologist Laura Bohannan in her classic novel, *Return to Laughter* (under the nom de plume of Eleanore Smith Bowen) which relates the life of an anthropologist doing field work with a primitive tribe in Nigeria, describes this quality.

> They knew how to live at close quarters with tragedy, how to live with their own failure and yet laugh . . . . Such laughter has little concern with what is funny. It is often bitter and sometimes a little mad, for it is the laugh under the mask of tragedy, and also the laughter that masks tears. They are the same. It is the laughter of people who value love and friendship and plenty, who have lived with terror and death and hate.

> To be worst,
> The lowest and most dejected thing of fortune,
> Stands still in esperance, lives not in fear;
> The lamentable change is from the best,
> The worst returns to laughter (1964, p. 297).

During the period of slavery, the black man learned that self-depreciating humor accommodated his master and was not offensive. It became a subtle way of ridiculing white concepts of black stereotypes: verbal difficulties, chicken stealing, fighting, freedom from sexual inhibitions, laziness, dishonesty. The Negro preacher and religious practices were also the butt of such humor. The use of humor as a technique in racial conflict has been described earlier. Since the Blacks were the first minority group to force Americans to deal with the issue of racial prejudice, the humor of the Black revolved in large measure around this issue. The humor became overt rather than convert, and anti-white jokes became more aggressive.

Particularly enjoyable to the Black is any incident or joke which shows Jim-Crow backfiring. The situations in which the Black is treated as a "darky" and then discovered to be the superior of the white in distinction, rank, or education are common. Some humor has a macabre flavor. The story is told of a black college president stepping off a train, who puts his arms out to catch a white woman behind him who has tripped. He suddenly realizes he is in Atlanta, drops his arms, and lets her fall. A study of jokes among university students (Middleton, 1959), comparing a southern white university with a Negro University in 1959, found that the Negro students told four times as many anti-Negro jokes as anti-white jokes.

The humor of today, post-civil-rights movement, still shows a need by Blacks to express hostility toward whites and to satirize themselves and their situation, but there is more openness and the humor is understood and enjoyed by the white man as well. The current literature describing the history and culture of the Blacks —the discrimination, and the problems, along with courses on Black studies — have assisted in this understanding and change.

In the literature on health and illness in the Black-American culture, one early study of cultural influences on patient behavior describes the use of humor by black patients in a southern hospital (McCabe, 1960, p. 13). Most of the patients were of low income status and poorly educated and did not seek medical care early. A lack of understanding of their illness was evident and they were obviously hesitant to ask for service or express dissatisfaction. One method attempted was through joking and humorous behavior. The problem was that the nursing staff missed the cues because they either resented it or did not understand the function of the behavior and only looked at it as "cute."

There is an element of suspiciousness and lack of trust on the part of the black patient which keeps him from using health care facilities until he is quite ill. He fears the prejudice, impersonality, and bureaucratization. The history of the health status of the Negro is directly related to his social status and social relations. As his status improved and his education, economical and social activities increased, so did his health status improve. In the past 60 years there has been a change from magical medicine to acceptance of the concept of disease and scientific medicine, although elements still remain. Many Blacks still seek as a first recourse the lay referral system: that is, pseudo- and para-medical healers, the fortune-tellers, mediums, herbalists, and makers of home remedies. Lack of funds and lack of sophistication with the health care system prevent many from seeking care. Preventive medicine for many is nonexistent, not from lack of awareness, but rather related to the general concept of future orientation. The body is just another object to be worn out and not repaired, to be enjoyed in youth and suffered and endured in old age. This concept changes as the Black becomes more middle class. For the many deeply religious Blacks, there is also an element of perceiving illness as a punishment.

Therefore one puts oneself in the hands of God and asks the minister to pray, rather than seeking medical care (Hines, 1972).

Leininger (1970) describes two situations in the care of the Afro-American patient. In one case, the black Southern male had difficulty trusting that the white nurse was really interested in caring for him since help and care given to the black people by the Southern whites is not common, especially by someone in a superior position. In the second situation, a black nurse who had been born and reared in the north, was uncomfortable taking care of a black male patient from the South. She noticed his mannerisms and language were different from hers and she did not want to be identified with these behaviors.

As with the Indian and Spanish-American cultures, there are variations in the black culture throughout the country and between various economic and status levels. Many patients resist seeking medical care because of the lack of understanding of differences in the diseases which affect them and the differences in care required.

In the study conducted by this author, many of these points were evidenced. One black professional, in an interview, felt Blacks use humor both to express hostility and to deal with the stresses. Some jokes with racial overtones, she said, can be shared with other minorities, but not with whites, and many jokes which would be denigrating if initiated by whites are tolerated within minority groups. Because of the cultureal paranoia, she felt most Blacks would be suspicious of any joke initiated by a white person, especially anything which might reflect stereotypes.

That Blacks do joke with each other about white stereotypes of them was described by one black aide with this joke:

> A black man who had been walking stopped outside a White mortuary. He was tired and asked if he could rest inside. He laid down on a table in a room with two dead bodies and fell asleep. The embalmer comes in and rolls all three tables into the embalming room. Later, he comes out and tells the boss all three bodies are done. The boss tells him there are only two! The embalmer replies: "There were three, two white and one black." The boss says, "But the black man wasn't dead!" The embalmer says, "You know, he kept trying to tell me that. But, then, you know how those Blacks lie!"

However, these "anti-Negro" jokes which satirize the stereotypes would not be told to the white man, this aide contended, because Blacks would never "put down" the black man in front of the white man; rather the humor used would get back at "Whitey." There are many jokes, she said, that are told in the black community that would be reversed so that the white man is the butt of the joke when told to a white man.

Some of this is changing, and in an atmosphere of trust and acceptance, the humor around racial differences can occur. Two examples of humorous incidents described by a white nurse in this study points this out.

> A young black male, waiting impatiently in the clinic to see the physician, joking with the nurse about not having to go through all that jive about checking in, said, "You know they call me J.J. [referring to the TV character in the show "Good Times."] I'm just like him." The nurse laughed and said, "You're better looking than J.J., but just as ornery!" The patient continued to mimic "J.J.s" manner of walking and talking, apparently enjoying the situation.

> Another black male patient, bundled to the ears in heavy coat, scarf, gloves, hat, and ear muffs, on a cold wintery day, began to slowly take off one piece at a time as he searched for his hospital plate to give to the clinic clerk. The nurse said, "You look awfully cold this morning." He said, "How can you tell?" She responded, "Cause your nose is red!" The patient laughed and all the other patients waiting behind him roared also.

Another example was reported by a white nurse caring for a black male patient following lung surgery. The patient was complaining about coughing all night and jokingly said he "thought he was coughing up sutures. Black, of course."

There were the same varied responses from the professionals when questioned as to whether there was a difference if the professional were a nonmember of that culture. Some said there was no difference, and several of the humorous incidents reported showed a good relationship that could have occurred in any nurse-patient interaction. However, there were those who felt there was a difference. The black culture has a language of its own, one nurse said, both literally and figuratively. Persons from the same culture can interact with each other in a soft joking way with language that would sound hostile if used by whites.

A black male patient waiting in the clinic to see the physician was complaining loudly, "I've been here two hours!" The black nurse's aide smiled and said, "I've been here four hours. What you complainin' about?" The patient laughed and settled down again to wait.

Although not related to health and illness per se, a book by an educator describing the problem of educating minority group, lower economic-level youngsters in our inner cities may serve to illustrate how an understanding of the culture makes a difference (Foster, 1974).

The youngsters used their streetcorner behavior to test their new, well-intentioned, middle-class teacher. Pupils walked in and out of the room, asking about reading comics, and getting off last period. Someone threw a crumpled-up piece of paper at the teacher. Thinking about his psychology courses which said, "Decontaminate through humor; make a joke out of things," the teacher said, "If that's the best you can do, you'd better hand it up!" Whereupon "all hell broke loose." The class set out to show him they could do better (p. 8).

The humor failed because the teacher did not understand that, in streetcorner behavior, one must always prove one's self physically, without a show of fear. It is a life style that courts violence and physical aggression. His pupils expected the same from him. Even black parents expect teachers to be tough disciplinarians and "make" their children learn. They view fear as prejudice!

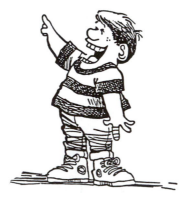

When the teacher began to understand the culture and the language, his style of humor changed and was effective. The students understood extroverted outgoing humor. "Acting crazy,"

"woofing," and "ribbing" helped: such behavior as hanging one youngster on a hook on the classroom door or jumping on the desk in "impassioned presentation." Often, the teacher would pick up a paper and read, "Wow — did you see this? John Frank was picked up by the police outside of the A&P on 125th Street for stealing a lollipop from a baby in a carriage." As the class laughed and howled, the teacher would note who was laughing the loudest and go on reading, inserting that youngster's name, "Jose Rodriquez was arrested for knocking over a Boy Scout helping an 80-year-old lady across the street" (p. 254).

Humor, to be effective, not only requires an acceptance and understanding of the cultural background, but also requires an atmosphere in which humor is acceptable and in which there is mutual trust and respect for each other. Of the total 29 humorous incidents, both observed and past recollections, 17 emanated from one unit, the surgical outpatient clinic of a large general hospital. This seemed to be the direct result of the atmosphere of that unit. The head nurse used humor with both patients and staff as a normal part of her interaction. She felt it was the only way she kept the staff able to cope with a hectic daily schedule of an average of 180 patients a day, often with some 20 physicians coming in and out. She used humor to control the situation, to give direction. When she needed to correct or admonish someone, she used "pet names" which set the frame for knowing "something was coming." When Albertine, the black desk clerk, became loud and noisy, the nurse would say, "OK, Albertooney..." or "Razzevelt" for the black orderly, Roosevelt. If the staff were madly dashing around, she might say, in passing, "If you're confused, maybe you need hormones!"

Since it was an inner city hospital, the patients who used this clinic came from all ethnic groups and cultures. The staff was also mixed. The head nurse was white, with three white, three black, and three Chicano staff. The head nurse felt that having staff of varied cultures was a distinct advantage in meeting their patients' needs. Very often "they can respond to each other in a language of their own."

In her interaction with patients, she had very carefully thought through her philosophy. "There needs to be respect and compassion and concern for the patient to use humor. The patient has to trust you and although sometimes the humor is rank, and you need to be direct and honest, you never make fun of or put the patient down. You catch his sense of humor!" She used humor to ease situations, but always came back to "concern."

> Many patients who come to the Clinic are elderly, economically in poor straits, often on fixed incomes. Yet, the hospital screening process requires that each time the patient must be asked if there is any change in income. The head nurse often says: "You haven't married a rich man since last time?" or "Found an oil well?" Then perhaps something like: "I know how hard it must be to manage today with this inflation."

> In teaching post-cast care to a patient with an extensive leg cast, she explains how to manipulate with it and then says, "Wait till you try to sit on the john!" This always gets a laugh! Then she goes on to explain how to support the leg when sitting.

Sometimes one must be alert to cues given by the patient that he is using humor to ease a situation.

> A chronic alcoholic with severe brain damage had obvious difficulty with his speech and thinking during the screening process. He could not seem to respond to a question regarding his address. An alphabet kept coming out rather than numbers. The nurse finally just moved on to the next question. "Nationality?" The patient smiled and said, "Well, I'm Polack." Both patient and nurse laughed.

The head nurse also gave an example of her humor that failed.

> An 80-year-old woman, with bleached blond hair, who always gave her age as somewhere between 47-55, consistently came in without an appointment and always wanted to be seen immediately. The nurse jokingly said, "Anyone as beautiful as you should be seen." The patient did not smile, rather she reacted negatively to the humor.

The humor hit too close to home: her obvious denial of reality, of her age and loss of beauty. There is always that fine line when teasing may become an insult.

# CONCLUSIONS

There is much more investigation and research to be done in this area, not only with these cultures but others as well. The results of this study cannot give us conclusive answers to the questions we have raised about humor and culture. Perhaps it has only raised more questions! When we describe a culture, are we accurately portraying a people, or are we portraying a stereotype? Are we describing characteristics which are a function of being poor rather than ethnic characteristics? What really constitutes an "American?"

The diversity of opinions expressed in this study suggests that there is a diversity within each culture or ethnic group, not only group or geographic differences but individual differences as well. The differences in the use of humor were related to the cultural beliefs, beliefs about health and illness, to the minority group's status, to the degree of acculturation and the socioeconomic status.

Therefore, the first basic assumption is that the cultural background of the patient must always be a consideration. The second assumption is that each person must then be assessed in terms of where he is within that culture. Here, a knowledge and understanding of that specific culture will be helpful in making this determination. The patient's degree of acculturation into Western culture must be evaluated. The Navajo from the reservation, the Chicano from the barrio, the Black from the ghetto have a different perspective compared to his counterpart who has attained middle- and upper-class status and a university education.

Most important to remember is that within all cultures there are changes in attitude. No longer do we find embarrassment or rejection, but rather a resurgence of pride in an ethnic heritage. Expression of this feeling ranges from a quiet display to an aggressive overreaction. Most individuals are simply incorporating the old and the new into a more comfortable way of life.

Just as the humor of a group or culture gives us clues to the function of that group, so the humor of each individual will reflect where he is in relation to his culture. And, of course, the degree of trust and respect and friendship established between patient and health professional will always make a difference in the degree and kind of humorous exchange which is acceptable.

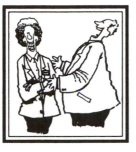

# 13
# Humor in Clinical Areas: An Update

Humor was identified in my earlier research as a significant therapeutic tool used in the health care system by patients and staff in managing the many stresses encountered. Further study was needed, not only to validate the functions and purposes for humor previously described, but to document and update what kind of humor was occurring.

Since direct observation of this large natural setting by an individual researcher is difficult and long-term, a collection of recalled and reported observations from health professionals over an eight-year period were analyzed (Robinson, 1988).

Some 1060 anecdotes were used, 840 were recalled humor and 220 were reported observations. These health professionals had attended my workshops, classes, programs, and speeches. Participants were asked to recall a favorite joke or funny personal story and a health care-related humorous incident as a pre-exercise and in some classes to analyze the effect as a post-exercise. As field work in six classes, students were asked to record observations of humorous incidents for a 2-week period. The observation guide developed in my original research was utilized by the participants. All these anecdotes were coded and analyzed. The favorite joke or personal funny story was analyzed as to type, whether it was health related, the kind of humor (situational, canned or practical joke), the style and the predominant theme. The health related incidents were analyzed also as to kind, style and theme: with whom the humor occurred, who initiated it, where it occurred (high stress or low stress areas), the target of the humor, and whether it was planned or unplanned. It was then analyzed for the sociological, psychological or educational purpose it served, the results or effects of the humor and in what clinical area it occurred (Research tools available from author).

These were 18 groups from mixed clinical backgrounds and five specialty groups. The groups varied in age from new graduates to the seasoned health professional. They came from all parts of the country, from the East Coast, the West, Hawaii, and from a wide variety of health settings.

There was a consistency in the kind of humor reported. Over the eight-year period there was an updating to current situation, technologies, and anxieties. For example, jokes about monitors and psychiatrists moved to cat scans, trauma centers, the aging population, and from Herpes to AIDS. There were similar "dumb" student stories. For example, the "vase" story reappeared. As I told the story, a student in the class shouted, "That happened to me, too!" The same "jokes" reappeared in different groups, in different parts of the country, with slight variations. The story of "That's God; He likes to play doctor!" reappeared with variations. As Freud said — a joke spreads across the country like "wild fire."

The limitations of "recalled" humor is that we have a tendency to remember only that humor which is extremely funny or those embarrassing ludicrous incidents which are recalled afterwards with hilarity. The everyday banter, witticisms, pleasantries, jocular talk, and "horsing around" is forgotten or lost in the daily activities. However, the large sample of both recalled humor and observed humor was statistically significant to support the assumption about the use of humor in health care, that humor as a communication tool has therapeutic value. It also supported the social and psychological functions described in my original research.

Asking the participants to recall their favorite joke, or story or the funniest thing that ever happened to them, was intended to establish the individual's sense of humor. Only 31% were health related. Some could not come up with one! The highest themes of humor were: incongruous/absurd/ludicrous (dumb, embarrassing incidents), sexual humor, and nonsense humor.

It was interesting to note that in the recalled health related anecdotes, the same three themes topped the list — incongrous, sexual, and nonsense humor, but with an increase in the scatological, gallows and hostile humor. In the reported observations, the gallows and hostile humor increased again as did nonsense humor, indicating that people bring with them into the health setting their usual humor preferences. But, because of the nature of this strange world of health care, where we deal with blood, guts, naked bodies, excrements, intimate activities, trauma, disabilities, crises, and death, the humor becomes relevant to the situation and the hostile, raunchy, and gallows humor emerges and increases as the stress level rises.

The style of the humor changed. In the recalled health care situations, ludicrous behavior (non-verbal pratfalls, getting splattered with blood or vomitus, stabbing yourself with a hypodermic needle) headed the list with verbal play, wit, clowning and jocular talk following. In the observed humor, jocular talk headed the list, with witticisms next. In recording humor as it happened, this humor is captured. And, in both recalled and observed health humor, the situational/spontaneous humor was high at 79-89%.

There was more humor recalled and observed in high stress areas (like O.R., E.R., Critical Care) with more gallows, hostile and sexual themes. In these areas there was more humor between staff rather than with patients. It was used to reduce the tension, ease the reality shocks and decrease burn-out.

In low stress areas (like medical-surgical and obstetrical units) more witticisms and jocular talk occurred. More humor between patients and staff occurred, with patients initiating slightly more humor than the staff. The use of humor by patients was primarily related to relief of anxiety, resolving social conflict and to lighten their tragic situations.

In the operating room, a high stress area, sexual humor predominated. (We have always known that if you wanted to hear the raunchiest jokes, you checked out the O.R.!). There is a need to laugh harder and to reduce the high tension. Sexual humor predominated rather than gallows humor because this area is more often one of hopeful outcome than death or negative outcome. Ludicrous behavior was also high (i.e., surgeons keep losing their tied surgical trousers!).

Overall, the highest category of purpose for the use of humor for both staff and patients was a relief of anxiety, stress, tension, and embarrassment (59.6% in both recalled and observed humor). Resolving social conflict was next highest, dealing with all those behaviors in our society considered taboo, which are expected to occur in health care without embarrassment. Other purposes included: outlet for anger, hostility, frustration (13.8%), social control (11.2%), group cohesion (10.9%), lightening heaviness (7.5%), establishing relations (6.8%), change (2.3%), denial (0.8%) and survival (0.5%). Only the predominate purpose for each incident was identified, but, obviously there is an overlap of psychological and social purposes.

For the large number of ludicrous situations which occurred for which no pre-determined purpose could be established, comic relief was the result. Comic relief/delight was the major result of 44.2% of the humor described, 42.7% expressed a feeling of relief from stress, 7.6% was used to establish rapport, 1.7% reported that persons reacted negatively to their humor, and 3.0% used the humor to facilitate expression of emotions and a serious discussion.

As was expected, 87.4% of the humor was unplanned, spontaneous and situational. Only 12.4% were a deliberate, conscious, planned use of humor through a practical joke, cartoon or telling of a joke or story or a planned witticism.

This study documented again that humor does occur in the health care setting, it does play a therapeutic role, and has value for both patients and staff. But, the need to increase the planned use of humor is apparent and gallows, sexual and aggressive humor needs to be recognized and accepted for its therapeutic role in high stress areas. It provides the balance needed to cope with the tragedies, crises, and unrelenting stress associated with the health care arena.

Another outcome of the eight-year study was the indication that humor does occur in all clinical settings. No area is devoid of humorous occurrences and laughter. Only the kind of humor will vary. There was an increase also in the reported use of humor in specialty areas like critical care, cancer units and hospice care, and in children's units, and care of the aged.

# HUMOR WITH CHILDREN

"Ask me why I have that light in my bed?

Why? "Cause I'm a light sleeper!"

Humor for the child is just as beneficial as it is for the adult. In the process of growing up, the child experiences many anxieties, fears, frustrations and disappointments, and many demands for adaptation to a sometimes threatening environment (Martin, 1989). The emotional impact of illness and hospitalization can elicit overwhelming traumatic and fear-producing stresses. The effect of hospitalization on the child can be viewed as similar to "visiting a newly-discovered planet" (D'Antonio, p. 267).

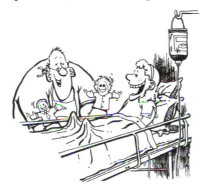

Coping with laughter and play is good mental health for the child as well as for the adult. Humor turns negative experience into positive ones (Wolfenstein, 1954). The ability to respond with humor and laughter in the face of adversity and to the stresses of growing up is an important skill in the child's repertoire of coping strategies (Martin, 1989).

Children's humor is closely related to play. Although playfulness is an ingredient in all humor, play, with laughter, is often the primary mode of expression of humor for the child. A child's humor is also related to his cognitive level and developmental level.

The development of the sense of humor parallels the intellectual, social, psychological and physical development of the child. As children master the developmental tasks of each stage of development, the humor emerges. Based on the psychodynamic model of the emotional, psychosexual development, Wolfenstein (1954) identified three stages in humor development: play, "jesting," when language begins, and use of the "joke facade" when the ability to conceptualize begins around age 6-7. McGhee (1979, 1980, 1983, 1989) developed his model from the "cognitive" experience and is linked to Piaget's stages of intellectual development. For an extensive review of humor development, see McGhee (1979, 1983, 1989), Honig (1988), and Pearson (1965).

How humor is expressed, then, depends on the child's age and development, but play and fantasy are the child's early way of coping with stresses. Children's creation of nonsense and absurdity and play is really aimed at reaffirming their belief that the world is organized and orderly, says McGhee (1979)! When the fantasy is recognized as not real, they can laugh at it and thus anxiety or aggressive feelings are reduced. Watching cartoons of the Road Runner and Bugs Bunny where someone is run over, blown up, pounded in the ground, but always "gets up" and survives, is "fantasy aggression." The child sees the incongruity, knows it is safe to have angry feelings, and releases them in the process of laughter.

A child's early attempts at humor are not what adults would find funny. As a matter of fact, many children's verbalizations which are amusing to adults are in fact mere mistakes of language or manifestations of innocence (Bariand, 1989). An example is the child who misuses words, who does not understand and misinterprets what he has heard or seen.

"Dennis the Menace," commenting on Mr. Wilson's forgetfulness, says, "He must have old-timer's disease."

The young child admitted to the hospital, hears the voice of the nurse calling him over the intercom system in this room. Finally, he responds tearfully: "What do you want, Wall?"

The elementary school child is asked by his mother what he learned from the AIDS education he had at school. "Well, I don't really know, but, I think we are supposed to buy condominiums and stay out of intersections."

Therefore, the adult or professional care-giver must be aware of what is fun and play and humor for the child. Respond to the child's use of humor. And, integrate play and fantasy and silliness and absurdity into humorous interventions with the child, always being certain that the child knows the care-giver is "playing."

The fears of the environment, the equipment, the medical treatments and laboratory testing can be diminished through use of dolls, teddy bears, toys, and other playful activities to "play out" the activity in educating and reassuring the child. Children rely on the use of fantasy and humor to reduce the tension and resolve conflict (D'Antonio, 1989). They will use their own fantasies or rely on others to "make them laugh" (Long, 1987). Professional clowns or staff utilizing "clowning" techniques can "poke fun" at the fearful routines, doctors, and treatments.

D'Antonio suggests taking a play history to provide insight into where to begin with play and humor activities, always being aware of the child's developmental level and age, but learning something about his past play behavior.

A discharge of emotional energy through physical play can be therapeutic. With older children, using joking, witticisms, cartoons, and practical jokes at their level can be an effective use of humor. School age children and adolescents will also use humor in return in response to their feelings about illness and hospitalization. An example is a 15-year old in a complete body cast who talked about a summer job for herself, "rolling down cement" (Wessel, 1975).

Children's humorous quips and play activities (use of drawings, telling stories) will reveal their fears and be a clue to the professional as to their needs. The use of humor in therapy with children can be used to enhance rapport and strengthen the relationship, enhance the child's ego strength, and self esteem, counter fear and anxiety and serve as a source of pleasure in the difficult process of therapy (Ventis, 1989).

Establishing a climate and special playrooms within the hospital and other care-giving areas produces an environment which is conducive to relieving stress but also fosters the child's use of humor as a coping device for growth and healing.

A "humor room" established at Children's Hospital, UCLA Harbor, includes a TV, cartoons, pictures of Yogi Bear on the wall, posters, games, stuffed animals, silly hats, and puppets to look like the doctors and nurses. "Christmas in July" parties and "Special Olympics," and clowns are events! The staff use themselves in the interactions with the children, deliberately making mistakes, telling stories on themselves, and playing jokes on each other.

Rivera (1988), a child life specialist in a child's "respite" center, utilizes funny hats, silly words, musical games, humorous books, magic "tricks" and a group joke book of the children's "Ha! Ha!'s." In lifting a patient, she may ask "what would you like to be today —a sack of potatoes or a bag of carrots?" In using humor with children she advises keeping it simple, use exaggeration, look for the laughable moment or movement and be open to the spontaneous unexpected time to add humor. For children, humor is a "warm fuzzy" of love.

Humor, D'Antonio says, requires an atmosphere of mutual respect and trust. "To reduce stress for children through the use of humor is an act of love" (1989, p. 168). McGhee (1989) summarizes with "keeping children in stitches with humor should help minimize the stress encountered while waiting for their stitches to be removed" (p. 264).

"What happens when ducks fly upside down? They quack up!"

# HUMOR IN AGING

There is much about old age, the last years of life, that can be painful: physical decline, chronic diseases and terminal illnesses. But the indication from the observation of the elderly, and the increased use of humor in society about aging shows that older people are ready to laugh at themselves! The use of humor by the elderly can reduce their anxieties, fears, depression, and pave the way to adaptation and acceptance of the limitations in the aging process. It gives them a hopeful perspective and the strength to survive.

Research on humor in the aging process has been meager until recently. *Humor and Aging*, edited by Nahemow, McCluskey-Fawcett and McGhee (1986), is the first to look at humor as a positive behavior. Much research has focused on the attitude toward aging as presented in jokes, stories and birthday cards. Most of the humor shows negative attitudes toward aging, with the themes related to age concealment, declining physical, mental and sexual ability, and changes in appearance and attractiveness (Palmore, 1986).

"You know you're getting old when everything hurts and what

doesn't hurt doesn't work."

"At my age, I don't even buy green bananas!"

However, with the elderly increasingly living longer and healthier, the joking is beginning to be more positive.

> The 90-year old mother admonishes her 60-year old daughter about her health and suggests she see her doctor and have a check-up. When the 60-year old daughter returns, the mother says, "Well?" The 60-year old daughter says, "The doctor says I'm just fine! As a matter of fact, I'll probably live to be a 110!" The 90-year old mother sits back, pensively, and then says, "Oh dear! What ever will I do with a 110-year old daughter!"

Not much research has been reported on the use of humor in the aged in related health care settings. Since the elderly often make up a large proportion of the patients in acute care facilities, and because people vary in their appreciation and use of humor, the humor may or may not be related to the aging process per se, but to the situation itself as seen in examples in previous chapters. However, the humor does occur.

> During a physical examination, an elderly patient pointed to her bosom and said, "Look, even these have wrinkles!"

An early survey of the use of humor in a nursing home (Jaeger & Simmons, 1970) aroused considerable controversy because it was not put in the context of humor in a broad sense, but the question was asked about using "kidding" or "joshing" with these aged ill and treating them as children! The end result was that suggestions for the positive use of humor emerged. "Poking fun" was not a mutually amusing situation, and teasing or humor carelessly bandied about could hurt rather than help.

Age does make a difference in the kind of humor used when there is an age gap between staff and patient. The elderly may feel the "younger" staff are being sarcastic. Humor should be used carefully, allowing for individual differences, the patient's state of well-being, and his ability to comprehend. Humor can bring warmth and cheer and raise the patient's self-esteem. It can provide a welcome relief from the monotony of the institution and show the patient that "someone cares. Humor becomes a saving grace for many of them" (Ibid, p. 57). The use of humor can allay many feelings of embarrassment and anger at their incapacity. One nurse shared that she had a joshing relationship with a dying incontinent patient in which mutual kidding about her need for work and his anxiety to see her employed helped both of them through innumerable bed changes which were a source of great dismay to him (Ibid, p. 63).

> An Activity Director in one nursing home trying to encourage an 80-year old resident to participate told her that she had heard all the excuses, the patient responded, "What if I told you I was pregnant!"

In a research study (Collins, 1988) carried out in a major New York nursing home where the climate of the institution was not attuned to the use of humor, the researcher found that humor was used as a mechanism by patients to cope with feelings of aggression, of powerlessness and loss of status when they were admitted to the nursing home. They believed they were deprived of control over their lives. Direct expression of their anger was considered inappropriate and could invite retaliation from those upon whom they depended. The residents used their humor to deride each other, the staff, certain aspects of institutional life and their relatives.

In 1978, The Andrus Volunteers of the Ethel Percy Andrus Gerontology Center of the University of Southern California became interested in the possibility that humor might be a therapeutic tool to improve the mental and physical health of residents in long-term care facilities. They developed a program of humorous activities and, as a result of their demonstration project, positive changes in the residents, including attitude change, more smiles and increased friendliness were observed. The residents increased their socialization, expressed more positive attitudes, became more open to participation. The report and guidelines for how to add humor to the climate were published in 1983.

Other reports of adding humor to the climate of the geriatric setting, have indicated a positive change in the sociability, alertness, and personal appearance of the patients.

Fry (1986) describes the physiologic value of laughter for the elderly who are bedridden or chair-bound, who cannot exercise, but who can laugh. "Mirth behavior provides exercise of greater or lesser degree." Cumulative laughter throughout the day may be significantly greater than that of an average marathon run, he says (p. 90).

In summary, the use of humor with the elderly has many beneficial effects, both emotionally and physically. We can only speculate whether humor is a factor in longevity, but it does increase the quality of that life. A look at famous, active, still functioning octogenarians reveals their positive outlook on life and feeling "young." When Picasso was asked by a friend why his later paintings had become more and more abstract and wild, almost "adolescent," he answered, "Easily. It takes a long time to become young!" (Kanin, 1978).

# SECTION 3
## CULTIVATING THE USE OF HUMOR

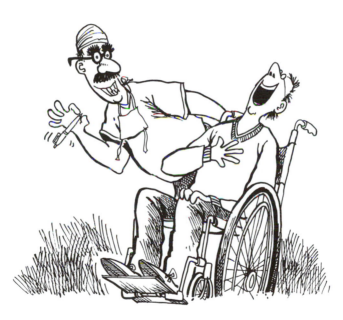

# 14
# Developing a Sense of Humor

We have been emphasizing the value of humor. We have shown that it is a form of communication which permeates our whole society, including the world of the health professional. We have also repeatedly voiced the opinion that not only must humor be understood, it also should be used as a deliberate therapeutic tool.

How does one go about cultivating that sense of humor, that humorous attitude, and incorporate the humor into the healing and health promoting process? I see four levels in achieving this goal.

The first level is the knowledge level (which we have attempted to do in the first two sections of this book). Just understanding a concept, its nature, its theories, functions and purpose can begin to make a change in behavior or application.

The second level is the acceptance level; the change in attitude, acceptance of the value of humor, and acknowledgement of its positive force. Just being open to the use of humor by others, feeling comfortable, and responding so the person does not feel rejected or put down when he may be using humor to cope with his stress is a first step. (Hopefully, you have achieved this level.)

The third level is a change in your own behavior, that is, developing or increasing your own sense of humor and, your humorous attitude. Recognize that humor is therapeutic and healthy for you personally as it is for your clients, and your increased humor will carry over into your professional life and practices.

The fourth and last level is the application level, or the change in your behavior with others. This is the ability to create humor, to utilize and create humorous situations and to make application to the care and health of your clients; to plan interventions with clients, and to add it to your communication with others and to the teaching process with students and peers.

"Fine!," you say, but how does one go about "cultivating" that humorous attitude and learning how to use humor consciously and effectively? Does that mean becoming a quipster? Building a repertoire of jokes? Becoming a clown? A practical jokester?

> I enjoy humor, but I've never been a joketeller, I can't even remember a joke.
>
> People say I'm funny, but I don't know why they laugh!
>
> Don't you have to be born with a sense of humor? You either have it or you don't!

These are typical reactions. The answer to all these questions is 'yes' and 'no'! No, because we should do only that which is comfortable for ourselves, that which suits our particular personalities, and fits our particular styles. Even a smile or a simple pleasantry can open doors and seem to create miracles.

And yes, humor can be cultivated and learned like any other skill or technique. There are many suggestions and techniques which can be learned and, with practice, become an integral part of one's pattern of communication.

> We regard the humorist, like the poet, as born, and not made, but this isn't quite true. Humor can be cultivated. It is made up of confidence, independence, boldness and observation (Hoffman, 1969).

However, just reading a book on humor, or reading humorous material, or committing oneself to practice humor is not enough. Nor is learning a series of devices for creating one-liners or jokes enough, in itself, although all of these are helpful in producing the end product.

Rather, the first necessary step is to analyze ourselves, and our own "sense of humor." Humor is first and foremost an attitude —almost an attitude toward life, a willingness to accept life and to accept ourselves "with a shrug and a smile," with a certain lightheartedness.

> To accept, in the end, existence, not because it's wonderful, not because it's divine, not because it's just or reasonable, or even satisfactory, but simply and plainly because it's all we've got (Mindess, 1971, p. 145).

Yet this is not a sense of resignation or even indifference, but rather a sense of mastery over life. D. H. Monro (1951) has called this a "god's-eye view." It implies the ability to be objective, to view the absurdity of one's plight and to be a free, detached observer of one's fate.

A precise definition of a "sense of humor" has never really been attempted. It usually includes this readiness and ability to laugh at ourselves, our own weaknesses, and to grant ourselves a degree of humanness, but it also implies an appreciation of humor as well as an ability to create humor and to "be funny." We often attribute a sense of humor to the person who is always laughing and smiling and "making jokes."

Eysenck (1972) refers to three different meanings to the sense of humor. If someone laughs at the same things as we do, that is the conformist meaning. If he laughs a great deal and is easily amused, that is the quantitative meaning. If he is the life of the party and tells funny stories and amuses others, that is the productive meaning. What we will be referring to in our use of the term sense of humor is an attitude which encompasses all of these meanings or dimensions, an attitude which senses the ludicrous and the absurdity of life, and which can be expressed in a variety of ways.

It is this "cosmic perspective" sense which Moody (1978) says is the "health-giving" value of mirth, the "ability to perceive life comically without . . . losing any love or respect for himself or for humanity in general" (p. 5). If we are to encourage this comic view of life's ups and downs in our patients, we must first achieve it in ourselves.

How does this attitude come about? Is it an instinctive quality, one with which we are born? Or is it a developmental process? Actually, most studies indicate that it is laughter or the smile which is considered genetic or biological, and the sense of humor, as we have defined it, is a developmental process, one which follows the course of normal physical, social, intellectual and emotional development; our sense of humor is influenced and learned through environmental influences (McGhee, 1979, Grotjahn, 1957). The ability to laugh is also related to the ability to play, to fantasize and to our capacity for tolerating ambiguity, incongruity and absurdity. The key to the development of humor and the kind of humor children use is related to the developmental tasks and cognitive intellectual level at each stage or age of the child. As children master these tasks humor evolves.

The smile is the first social response of the infant which phylogenetically evolved from the startle reflex and has developed in man into a pleasurable reaction of small and pleasant stimulus changes. Rene Spitz (1946) in his famous study showed that the baby must see the full face and both eyes of the mother in order to respond. When the mother turns away, the smile disappears. Within the first 36 hours of life, the infant is capable of discrimination and imitation of facial expressions — including sticking out one's tongue! The implications are that the contact, cuddling, and playing by a mother fosters the smiling-laughter response. The earlier the smile, the earlier the laugh, and the more advanced the development. With his smile, the infant establishes himself as a human and a social being. The inability to smile demonstrates emotional starvation and loss of human contact.

The smile of the infant develops into the laughter of the baby. Play activity between adult and child in this early period consists of gross motor activities like tickling, bouncing, tossing in the air, chasing, and peek-a-boo. The baby's first reaction is startle and surprise which quickly turns to broad smiles and shrieks of laughter. The laughter is an expression of pleasure in the physical contact, as well as relief from the initial alarm. This same element of surprise remains in adult humor with the corresponding burst of laughter that follows the punch line.

When the child begins to talk, this gross motor humor gives way to verbal humor. Rhyming words and play with words, and displacement of words that have to do with toilet functions and the genitals, produce laughter in the two- to three-year-old. As he begins to master bodily movements — i.e., walking, toilet-training and other coordinated activities — his laughter is a response of superiority to these anxiety-producing situations. He laughs at the clown's clumsiness and antics and at involuntary or imitated flatus. The "belly laugh," says Grotjahn, stands halfway between the socially accepted noise of laughter and certain toilet noises which are taboo in company (1957, p. 75).

At four years of age, fantasy and imaginary playmates are characteristic of play, and humor is aroused by anything that is strange and unusual and "funny." The humor becomes silly and boisterous. There is name-exchanging and name-calling and wild laughter. There is a beginning interest in pictorial expressions of humor which show distorted figures or "funny" scenes and lead to an increased interest in "the comics."

At age five, the child begins showing an interest in games, which indicates a desire to playing together rather than the self-contained play of earlier years. The playing of cowboys and Indians, circus, house, cops and robbers consumes hours of time. This imaginative play, combined with a beginning formalization of intellectual behavior. produces the "riddle" as a pleasurable activity.

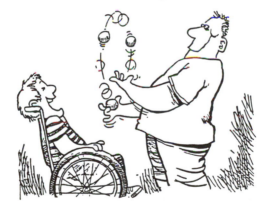

The riddle moves into the anecdotal joke at age six where there is a marked increase in verbal humor. The six-year-old suddenly develops a lusty interest in adult jokes and begins to develop a repertoire. Riddles and April-fool jokes and "moron" jokes are associated with a new interest in learning and in the issue of being smart or dumb. William Fry feels there is a transition at this age related to a beginning ability to abstract and conceptualize. This capacity is an essential ingredient in getting the point of a joke (1963, p. 14).

From eight to ten years of age, the child makes attempts to create his own humor through practical jokes and punning. He may repeat "dirty jokes" which he does not always understand. The ten-year-old's jokes may not seem funny to adults but to him it is an attempt to play with ideas and words. This is also a period when there is a laughing at the misery and misfortunes of others, i.e., the fat man and the man who slips on a banana peel, an indication of an ego strong enough to disguise aggression in a socially acceptable way.

A more outward display of aggressive humor occurs in the pre-adolescent. Slapstick comedy, clowning around, poking fun, and hurling insults are the signs of a more direct use of aggression, but are consistent with the early rebellion against authority of the 10- to 14-year-old.

By 16, there is a more adult level of abstraction, and an understanding of subtle implications and double meanings in jokes and cartoons. There is an interest in how jokes are told: timing, wording, and skill. Real humor, some authors feel, does not appear until adolescence. The adolescent begins to develop a sympathy for others and his "laughing at" begins to decline. He can use humor positively to "kid" a friend or to respond to criticism with kidding. And, he attempts to create humor. When I asked my 16-year-old daughter to tell me a joke going around in her circle, she said, "We don't tell jokes. We make them!" At a meeting of the youth group of the church, everyone who made a pun or witticism was finally fined five cents, so that the group could get on with the business at hand.

The development of a sense of humor thus parallels the development of the use of language and of thought; of the ability to reason and to conceptualize. Mature humor is the final integration of all these stages and also signifies an emotional maturity. The social, intellectual, and physiological tasks have been mastered. This mature humor is based upon deeper life experiences, and kindly, tolerant acceptance of oneself and therefore of others. A free and periodic regression to the enjoyment of the child-like humor of the comic, the clown, and slapstick comedy occurs and is possible because the energy is no longer needed for repression. The development of this mature or even "greater" humor described by McDougall, Freud and Maslow may go on long into adulthood.

What fosters the development of this sense of humor throughout childhood? Some authors suggest it may be the loving atmosphere in the home and school, freedom and opportunity to express oneself, and the experience of successfully coping with frustrating and anxiety-producing situations through humor. The modeling of the use of humor and frequent laughter by parents in the home is another consideration since children learn by imitation and identification. Humor can also be squelched by a rigid, serious environment. "That's not funny!" "Wipe that smile off your face!"

We can describe the normal, general course of the growth and development of a human being physically, socially, emotionally, and intellectually. Yet we know that each individual, based upon his experiences, develops his own unique combination of traits and characteristics, his own personality and behavior, which sets him apart from everyone else in the world. Similarly, with the development of a sense of humor, each person develops his own distinctive pattern. What he finds funny, how he reacts to humorous situations, how he makes use of humor, as well as his ability to create humor and "be funny," may be quite different from the next person's.

There is the view also that personality and a sense of humor are closely related and are not independent of each other. Goethe once said, "Men show their character in nothing more clearly than by what they think laughable."

Many studies have focused on the relationship of personality to a sense of humor or humor preference. The evidence is not conclusive, but a summary of these studies may provide a beginning understanding of the complexity of the relationship.

Several early studies indicated that extroverts preferred orectic (aggressive and sexual) jokes while introverts preferred cognitive (complex-clever) jokes, and that extroverts prefer derisive, superiority humor while introverts preferred nonsense, fantasy types of humor. This indicates that a person's typical personality or behavior extends to his preference in humor.

Aggression seems to be one trait which has attracted much study. Perhaps this is so because of the difficulty many persons have in accepting the relationship. Some studies demonstrated that enjoyment of humor led to a decrease in aggressive feelings. However, another study, which contradicts the cathartic effect of aggressive humor, found that angry female subjects were more aggressive following aggressive humor. Another research study questioned under what conditions one person's aggression toward another was judged to be funny. The investigators discovered that social perception was important. A good person's hostile act is seen as more humorous and less hostile. A victim who "deserves" the hostility he receives elicits more humor than an undeserving victim. Martin Grotjahn (1971), discussing the sexual joke, suggests that the discharge of aggression through laughter may facilitate the free and joyful acceptance of sex.

Humor tests have been devised over the years based upon these personality factors through the appreciation of various types of humor. These informal tests use jokes and cartoons catagorized by type, e.g. sexual, aggressive, nonsense and philosophical, to assess an individual's preference (Eysenick & Wilson, 1975; Mindess, 1971; Psychology Today, 1978). Mindess, et al (1985) further developed this concept. The Antioch Sense of Humor Inventory uses a broader range of humor types and includes questions and exercises to assess your own creativity and feelings about humor. The jokes and cartoons expand to include, besides the four basic types — nonsense, sexual, philosophical and hostile — social satire, jokes demeaning to men, jokes demeaning to women, ethnic, sick jokes and scatalogical (toilet) humor, on a scale from five (very funny) to one (not at all); or? if you don't understand the joke.

Examples:

1. Q. What does a grape say when you step on it?
   A. Nothing. It just gives a little wine.

2. It is better to keep your mouth shut and appear stupid than to open it and remove all doubt?

3. A farmer is showing a beautiful lady visitor around his farm. They watch a bull lustily mating a cow. Putting his arms around the lady's waist, the farmer says, "Boy, I'd sure like to do something like that." "Well, why don't you?" she replies. "It's your cow."

4. It's not what you don't know that hurts you. It's the things you know for sure that aren't true.

Our strong preference for one of these or groups, tells us something about our personalities and our "sense of humor." Look at what kinds of humor we like or detest or wince at? Do we enjoy subtle sexual, but not demeaning or gross sex jokes?

Mindess speaks to the rating problems which beset this kind of research in humor. Since our individual spontaneous humor varies from time to time and situation to situation, the moment of the testing may be reflective of our emotional state at the time. It is also difficult to compare a joke heard previously to a new joke. One joke may seem clever, but not laughable, whereas another moves the listener to laugh but is gross and not clever. What is important, however, is to note that we do indeed have a preference and that, by pursuing this notion, we can discover something interesting about ourselves.

Weighing whether we laugh because we are comfortable with that emotion or quality, or because we have a problem with it, or, on the other hand, whether we do not laugh because it is no problem or too much of a problem, creates some of the difficulty in analyzing the reaction scientifically. Other problems relate to the salience or relevancy of the topic. A single person who has no mother-in-law may not laugh at mother-in-law jokes. But he may laugh at the cleverness of the joke, even though he has no personal hostility toward mothers-in-law. Most of us fall into the category of enjoying some of each type of humor and disliking some of each.

The second part of the Antioch Sense of Humor Inventory asks our favorite joke; how do you rate your sense of humor, and have you ever used humor to cope with a situation? It also asks you to create humor by putting your own captions on cartoons, ending a sentence with something funny, like: "The world today . . .": to fill in a plaque on "Advice to Worried Lovers . . . ." or a sign: "Today's Sermon . . . ." and to write a funny inscription for your tombstone (p. 19-24).

This last part will also tell us something about ourselves and our sense of humor, i.e. are they self-directed, other-directed or at everyone and what themes keep reappearing. These are also exercises which can be used to increase our creativity — to learn to "think funny."

Tests to measure generalized individual differences in humor production and appreciation rather than preferences for particular types of humor were developed by Svebak (1974), *Sense of Humor Questionnaire*, and by Lefcourt and Martin (1986), the *Situational Humor Response Questionnaire.*

Svebak's test was concerned with the way the individual expressed or experienced humor. Respondents were asked to agree or disagree on a 1-4 scale to statements like:

I can usually find something comical, witty, or humorous in most situations.

People who tell jokes to make others laugh really do it to assert themselves.

I often find myself laughing in situations where laughter is quite out of place.

I feel that humorists often open my eyes to aspects of life that I seldom think about.

Lefcourt and Martin give situations and ask the respondent to imagine themselves in the situation and choose the phrase that best describes their reaction.

If you were eating in a restaurant with some friends and the waiter accidentally spilled a drink on you:
   a. I wouldn't have found it particularly amusing.
   b. I would have been amused, but wouldn't have shown it outwardly.
   c. I would have smiled.
   d. I would have laughed.
   e. I would have laughed heartily.

If you arrived at a party and found that someone else was wearing a piece of clothing identical to yours:
   a. I wouldn't have found it particularly amusing.
   b. I would have been amused, but wouldn't have shown it outwardly.
   c. I would have smiled.
   d. I would have laughed.
   e. I would have laughed heartily.

How would you rate yourself in terms of your likelihood of being amused and of laughing in a wide variety of situations?
   a. my most outstanding characteristic
   b. above average
   c. about average
   d. less than average
   e. very little

Another way to look at our "sense of humor" which may be more realistic is to make an ongoing analysis of our everyday reactions to humor and our own humorous creations. The spontaneous witticisms we come up with, as well as our day-to-day reactions to our personal situations, may be more revealing of our natural use of humor than formal tests.

The importance of the information we obtain regarding our humor in relationship to our own personalities is to use it simply as a guide to our own sense of humor, being aware of the situation in which it occurs, the frame of mind we are in, and our emotional state at the time. If we gain some clue as to the general state of our sense of humor and a clue to the style of humor with which we are most comfortable in keeping with our individual personalities, we can then look to the obstacles blocking the further development of our humor and to the frame of reference in which our sense of humor needs to be cultivated and expanded.

To begin to expand our humorous attitudes we need to allow ourselves the freedom to laugh; to begin to look for the absurdities in life — to put more playfulness into our lives. Mindess (1972) provides us with some guidelines. So many restrictions have been placed on us as children in the process of growing up that, as adults, we are wrapped in our own security blanket and have lost the ability to be spontaneous and genuine. He says the spirit of disruption and the exhilaration which the baby feels as he flies through the air can be rediscovered if we let humor help us to escape from the ruts of our minds and our self-imposed prisons.

The first step to acquiring a lively sense of humor is a readiness to "slip loose from organized modes of being" (p. 41). We must be willing to revel in utter foolishness: be impulsive, irreverent, and unashamedly childish. Laughter must be fed on awareness of the eternal human comedy. We must free ourselves from the bonds of conformity and "become elastic with regard to society's demands" (p. 41). We should allow ourselves to challenge all the shibboleths by which we live and we will rediscover the exuberance we knew as children. This release through humor, however, must be brief and our conventional view of life must be repeatedly re-established so that we can enjoy release from it again and again.

We must foster the conditions which help us to become nonconformists whose motto is "nothing sacred;" to dislodge our feelings of inferiority, modify our moral inhibitions, indulge in foolishness, break loose from habitual behavior, renew our playful spirits, and escape our inescapable conceit. Above all, Mindess says, the cultivation of humor requires that we learn to thrive on change.

None of these conditions is as easy to develop as they sound, because they conflict with our needs to be dignified, competent and superior creatures. However, if we believe that humans have the capacity to change, to continue to learn, and to change behavior, then we must believe that, even in adulthood, we can continue to develop, cultivate, and change our sense of humor. If we could not so believe, then all educators and human behavior professionals should simply "fold up their tents and silently slip away." We can teach an old dog new tricks and we can cultivate a sense of humor!

What it boils down to, again, is that a sense of humor is an attitude — an attitude that allows us to see the absurdity in life, in events and situations, in others, and in ourselves. How we express this attitude becomes an individual matter. Some of us are a Bill Cosby, others of us are a Don Rickles, and some of us are a Gracie Allen. This attitude of being "in fun" as Eastman calls it, is the foundation or framework we must cultivate in ourselves as a base for learning comedy techniques, utilizing humorous materials and exercises for expanding our humor, and, then incorporating humor into our professional practice.

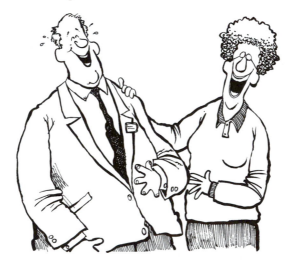

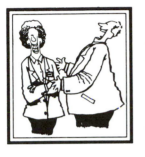

# 15
# The
# Techniques
# of Comedy

*Creating humor is like asking how to capture happiness. It is elusive,
subjective, and inexplicable. You know it when it's there and you can
feel its absence.*

Gene Reynolds
Coproducer, M\*A\*S\*H

How does one create humor? What makes it funny? This has
been one of the eternal questions surrounding the concept of
humor. Many theorists have responded as Gene Reynolds did, for
there is that quality of uncertainty, intangibleness, and subtlety in
humor. William Fry refers to it as a "paradoxical abstraction." We
never really know if we have achieved the right balance, the right
nuance, the right spark, until we hear that burst of laughter. Like
happiness, the harder we try to be funny, the more it escapes us.

Yet when pressed to define those elements, guidelines, and
techniques which one pursues in producing comedy, comedy
writers are able to do so, as does Gene Reynolds, in describing the
production of M\*A\*S\*H.

Comedy is lighter, smoother, more rhythmic than drama. One must avoid sobering assaults, long pauses, tight closeups and strain . . . look for the smoothness, surprise, subtle gestures and the eccentric . . . and, above all, the recognizably human behavior must be painfully honest. When you can teach an actor the difference between playing dramatically angry and comically angry, you are warm (Excerpts from a personal letter, September 23, 1975).

Reynolds has described, very succinctly, the core elements in the creation of humor: the right timing, the smoothness, the subtlety, the surprise, the absurdity, and the human factor.

Humor which points out some very familiar human dilemma or weakness which "strikes home" will produce the laughter of recognition and acquiescence. Charlie Chaplin attributed his success in making people laugh to a knowledge and study of human nature. In his classic article on comedy, George Meredith (1877) conveys this same thought: ". . . to touch and kindle the mind through laughter demands, more than sprightliness, a most subtle delicacy" (p. 206). The humorist must be "subtle to penetrate," and there must also exist a corresponding acuteness to welcome him.

The life of comedy is in the idea. As with the singing of the skylark out of sight, you must love the bird to be attentive to the song, so . . . you must love pure comedy . . . . And to love comedy you must know the real world . . . (Ibid, p. 210).

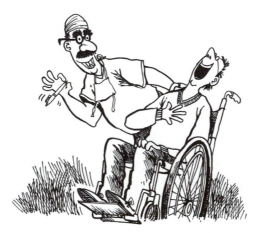

In more concrete terms, Sam Levinson suggests finding chuckles in the commonplace. Seek the common denominator in little things like television and dieting, and exaggerate it a bit. Robert Orben directs us to "think funny" and the comedy will "burst out in all directions" (1972). For "humor to work," he says," it has to cut to the heart of an issue or problem. It covers a kernel of truth, or perceived truth, with a coating of laughter" (Orben, 1988).

However, an attitude (which is what we are describing) must be practiced and developed if it is to become an integral, spontaneous aspect of our philosophy, view of life, and communication pattern. Furthermore, that practice must be a deliberate, conscious effort, often overpracticed and exaggerated, in order to be learned. There are a number of authors, joke writers, comedy writers and comedians who contend that humor can be cultivated, and have described in detail how to create humor (Orben, 1963, 1971, 1988; Adams, 1968; Whitney, 1969; Helitzer, 1984; Allen, 1987). Although their books are more in the realm of "how to" and for professional comedians, they nevertheless offer ideas for the would-be humorist in the health field. These guidelines for jokes, stand-up comedy routines, and one-liners may not always be appropriate for our own style of humor or for the quiet, simple pleasantries and situational humor which often occur in the health setting, but they do give us the essence of creating humor which is helpful in developing that quality of lightheartedness of "thinking funny," of the "god's eye view." In addition, they give us some tangible methods to practice, rather than just exhortations to "be funny," that allows us to incorporate humor in a more calculated fashion in our communication patterns, in our teaching practices, and in interventions with patients.

# THE BASIC ELEMENTS

Creating humor is somewhat like using a recipe to create bread: there are certain ingredients that must always be present if we are to achieve a recognizable product. However, there are modifications of these ingredients, and the addition of numerous other ingredients can create variations of the same product. There is also a distinctive pattern for blending the ingredients. There must be the right temperature and the right timing for cooking it. Finally, the end result, to be fully appreciated and enjoyed, must be served in an appealing fashion to just the right audience.

So with humor to be effective there are at least two basic ingredients which must be present, with many variations and many other ingredients which can be added. Humor must be blended in just the right way, in the right atmosphere, with the right timing, and presented with elegance and smoothness to the right audience.

The two basic ingredients of humor which seem always to be present in some degree are surprise and absurdity. There must be some unexpected twist which creates a shock of surprise; that surprise must be absurd or ludicrous, yet fit into the general context of the story or concept. We must be led down one corridor of thought and suddenly jolted into another by some unexpected turn of events. There are many variations of this surprise and absurdity but, like flour and liquid, both are there in some form and to some degree.

The many modifications and additional ingredients are elements which include incongruity, contrast, conflict, misunderstandings, play on words, double meanings, allusions, exaggerations, overstatements, understatements, fantasy, and sheer nonsense.

Let us look at some examples. There is a cartoon of a man with an arrow through his chest leaning over the receptionist's desk in a doctor's office. The nurse looking at the appointment book, is saying, "How about a week from Tuesday?"

The surprise response and incongruity of the desperate patient and the casual nonchalant nurse is so absurd, we have to laugh! The cartoon also points out a familiar frustrating situation: having to wait to see the doctor. But the contrast here is so sharp, it is funny rather than annoying.

The humor must also "fit" to be amusing. If the nurse had simply said, "The doctor is not in," it would not have been humorous at all. The incongruity concept must be a sudden perception of two obviously incompatible ideas, meanings, emotions, objects, situations, or events.

The double-meaning ingredient can be shown by this story, attributed to Lewellyn Thompson, Ambassador to Russia in the sixties:

> A Russian peasant is trudging down the road on a cold bitter morning when he sees a bird lying on the side of the road, half-frozen. In sympathy, he picks up the bird, holds it in his hands and tries to warm it. Spotting a freshly dropped, still warm pile of manure nearby, the peasant places the bird down

in the middle of the pile, and goes on his way. Responding to the warmth, the bird gradually thaws out and feeling good, he begins to chirp and sing. A wolf, not far away, looking for his morning breakfast, hears the singing, comes trotting over, pounces upon the helpless bird who cannot extricate himself, and eats him.

The moral of this story is, it is not always your enemies who put you in it, nor your friends who pull you out, but when you are up to your neck in it, for God's sake — don't sing!

We are led along with the story to a blank wall when the bird is eaten. So what's funny? Then, with a surprise twist, the story is turned into a moral with a double meaning attached. The absurdity, yet the direct "fit," of the moral makes us laugh.

Shaggy dog stories are another variation which are so unexpected and so nonsensical, they strike us as funny: "Why do you have that celery stuck behind your ear?" "Because I didn't have any lettuce."

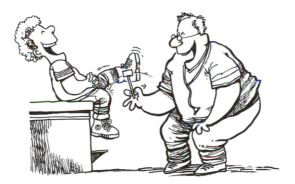

A play on words — puns, mispronunciations, and malapropisms — create humor. They are surprising and ludicrous. A patient referred to the Obstetrical Unit as the Obstruction Clinic, or called the Intensive Care Unit the "Expensive" Care Unit.

Exaggeration is an element dear to the heart of Americans, and especially to Texans.

A fellow walks into a bar in Texas and orders a beer. The bartender places in from of him a huge 2-foot glass, and says, "Everything in Texas is big." As the stranger sits there drinking his beer, a tall Texan walks into the bar. The stranger

gasps and asks, "How tall are you?" "I'm 7' 4", replies the
Texan, "everything in Texas is bigger." And, so it went.
Finally, after all that beer, the stranger asks for direction to the
rest room. He is told to go down the hall to the door on the left.
However, in his state of inebriation, he opens the door on the
right and falls into the swimming pool! He flounders and
gasps, and as he is struggling to get to the side, he keeps
yelling, 'DON'T FLUSH!!!'

The surprise ending, the ludicrousness of the situation, yet the
obvious fit to the concept of "big" is vividly demonstrated.

In addition to the basic ingredients, there must be a proper sequence and blending of those ingredients in order for the joke or humor to occur. The punch line must be held in abeyance and pre
sented in such a way that the surprise is created and the point is
made.

In the comic-strip, *The Family Circus*, one of the boys is reading
a joke book. He says,

"Wanna hear a joke, Dolly?"

"Uh-huh!"

"Okay, how does a witch tell time?"

"I don't know — how?"

"She wears a WITCH WATCH!"

Dolly gleeful, says as she dashes off to the other room,

"I'm going to tell that one to Daddy!"

"Daddy, do you know how a witch tells what time it is?"

"She looks at a clock, I suppose."

"No, she wears a watch on her wrist!"

Daddy does not laugh and looked perplexed, as Dolly runs off
crying.

"Daddy didn't laugh at my joke!"

Dolly flubbed the punch line and the whole point of the joke
was gone.

The proper sequence of events leading up to the punch line
should also contain those points to which the punch line refers. The
use of pauses, intonations, and gestures can also highlight the

crucial points. A dialect should be used only if the individual can do so with finesse, but can add to the effect of the story.

Proper timing is essential to the success of humor. It must occur at just the right moment. Many a witticism in a discussion or conversation gets a louder laugh than the content itself would indicate, simply because it "fits" so well and strikes the right note. The pace or tempo is also crucial to the build-up of the suspense when a joke is being told. The punch line must catch the listener unaware — and ready — not lost in boredom along the way. Proper timing also implies an appropriateness to the situation; that is, the atmosphere must be conducive to that bit of levity.

To round out the basic elements of a humorous undertaking, the neatness or the "elegance" with which the sally is delivered is vital. The humor must flow smoothly. If the humorist stumbles, loses track, hems and haws, he has lost it. Sometimes a spontaneous witticism can save the occasion and is funnier than the planned story.

> At a national conference, the chairman of the meeting was telling a story and suddenly couldn't remember the punch line. The audience giggled as she hesitated, and said, "Oh dear, I've forgotten the punch line." Then, she recovered her composure and said, "You know, the brain is really a marvelous thing. It starts working the moment you awake in the morning, and only stops when you open your mouth in front of an audience." That brought down the house!

A little later when a friend reminded her of the punch line to her story and she relayed it to her audience, it was no longer funny. It was out of context, the timing was off and the surprise element was gone.

Needless to say, the content of the humor is another crucial factor. Knowing your audience is the first prerequisite. Jokes about education to educators, about nursing to nurses, are more effective than those same jokes would be to business leaders or politicians. Effectiveness, says Mindess (1971), depends on the strength of the drive it releases in the listener. If it evokes a gut reaction, reduces anxiety, is not too gross and touches us where we live, it will be enjoyable (p. 167-168).

Max Eastman (1936) sums up the basic elements for serious

joke-makers in his "Ten Commandments of the Comic Arts;" although the language is quaint, it still conveys the essence of our previous discussion (pp. 290-326).

| Commandments | Interpretation |
|---|---|
| Be interesting. | It must arouse an emotional interest. |
| Be unimpassioned. | Don't crack jokes around topics about which people feel too intensely. |
| Be effortless. | Don't try too hard to be funny. |
| Remember the difference between cracking practical jokes and conveying ludicrous impressions. | A practical joke is a witty joke, brief, with the fun in the punch line or the "nub," while a ludicrous impression is a humorous story which can be spun out and is amusing all the way through. |
| Be plausible. | Successfully lead the audience on. |
| Be sudden. | Save the punch line and make it a genuine surprise. |
| Be neat. | A joke with a point that gets across. |
| Be right with your timing. | It has to be sprung. |
| Give good measure of serious satisfaction. | Jokes must amuse the audience. |
| Redeem all serious disappointments. | If the joke falls flat, redeem it by another funny comment. |

# STEPS TO BECOMING A HUMORIST

You are ready now to be a humorist, you say; where do you go from here? You have the right attitude, you understand the basic elements of a joke, now what?

### Step One: Choose your weapon: your style

Joey Adams (1968) suggests that we must choose our weapons, that is, find out what style is funny and comfortable for us. Do we see ourselves as a wit, a kidder, a humorous story teller, gag man, a joke-teller, a punster, a clown, a satirist, or a floater? Choose that comedy style, study that style, collect materials, and practice.

Each of these styles refers to a kind of humor. Generally, the average person enjoys and utilizes many varieties of humor, but some individuals, in keeping with their unique personalities, favor one variety over the other. If you find in your own analysis that one style seems to be your forte, recognize it and develop it. Who is your favorite comedian? Check out his/her style.

A research study which investigated the relationships between different types of comedians and their audiences compared Bill Cosby and Don Rickles (1973). Cosby makes us laugh at bits of human behavior common to us all. He pokes fun at our fallacies, but is never hostile or confronts us directly. Rickles, on the other hand, picks on his audience: 'Hello, dummy.' He makes fun of us and exposes our foibles. The subjects viewed Cosby as a nice guy, funny and harmless. They laughed at Rickles only if they were with a group of friends. Group solidarity was important: I'll laugh, if you will.

### Step Two: Collecting materials — base line data

Before we are ready to create on our own, developing a file of humorous materials will assist us not only in creating new jokes, but as an adjunct and resource base. Incorporating humorous material of others into our communications, conversations, lectures, speeches, and writings is an effective tool which we should always use even when we find ourselves becoming more spontaneous and creative.
1. Make a file of jokes.
2. Jot down amusing anecdotes and humorous situations.
3. Listen for witty remarks others make.
4. Jot down humorous signs, TV gags.
5. Record personal humorous experiences.
6. Collect boners, and newspaper funnies.
7. Save cartoons and magazine humor.
8. Collect comedy records and humorous poems.
9. Collect materials of comedians and comedy writers.

### Step Three: Creating your own humor

The gimmicks and techniques which comedy writers use to create the humor they produce can be used by the new humorist. There are four approaches or methods:
1. Tell second-hand jokes or stories.
2. Share humorous experiences of your own and others.
3. Modify old jokes, quips, and stories.
4. Invent or create new humor by using humorous devices.

The first two approaches are self-explanatory and the techniques for the right timing, the appropriateness, and methods of delivery have been previously described. However, the gimmicks to practice for three and four are presented in outline form with examples attached.

A. **Devices for modifying old jokes, quips, stories, gags, quotations, etc.**

  1. **Switching:** Dress up an old joke in new clothes. Make them fit the situation.

   "I don't fly on account of my religion — I'm a devout coward."

   One frog says, "I've got a man in my throat."

   "Old doctors never die — they just cut-out."

   "Old psychiatric nurses never die — they go into administration."

   "He who hesitates will hear horns tooting."

  2. **Personalize and localize:** Substitute name of place, city, person, or group to whom you are telling the joke, story, or anecdote. Relate a joke as an actual incident involving someone well known to your audience.

   A nursing leader discussing the discordancy and divisiveness in the profession, quipped, "What nursing needs is its own Henrietta Kissinger."

  3. **Poke fun at yourself:** Audiences love to feel superior. Make jokes about things that are happening to you. Using yourself as the butt of the joke makes you human and endears you to your audience.

   Following a "boo-boo" you've made: "Do you ever feel like you're in the wrong profession?"

B. **Humorous devices for creating humor.**

  1. **The humorous catalogue:** The injection of a humorous item into an otherwise serious list.

   "A politician on the campaign trail must be articulate, diplomatic, knowledgeable, have stamina and the digestion of an ostrich."

  2. **Exaggeration:** So overstate a truth as to make it absurd, yet leave the original idea obvious.

   "That room is so small, when you lie down the door knob gets in bed with you."

   "My nursing instructor was so old, she didn't teach history, she remembered it."

3. **The double-cross:** Wreck a plausible train of thought by an incongruous one and produce a shock of surprise.

"He was determined to stay alive, even if he died in the attempt."

"There once was a professor who dreamed he was lecturing and woke up to find it was true."

4. **Anti-climax:** A sentence or passage in which the ideas at the close fall off in dignity or importance.

"Our next speaker needs no introduction. He didn't show up."

"Now a quote from that famous child psychologist — our teenage babysitter."

5. **The insult:** Be sure of your gag and your audience.

"Hello, dummy."

Groucho Marx introducing a film: "Every once in a while Hollywood makes a great movie. Unfortunately, this isn't one of them."

6. **Nonsense-fantasy-escape from reality:** Gags are completely irrational and fantastically ridiculous.

Dog 1. "I feel so poorly."
Dog 2. "Have you thought of going to a psychiatrist?"
Dog 1. "Heavens, no! You know I'm not allowed on couches."

7. **Understatement:**

"If you can keep your head when all about you are losing theirs, maybe you don't understand the situation."

Cartoon: Trapeze artist fails to catch his partner, says "Oops, sorry."

Cartoon shows a fisherman in a rowboat on a lake, clutching a monstrous fish which is bigger than he is. Another man is rowing by and says "Had any luck?"

8. **Irreverence:** Poking fun at pomposities, lampooning authority and stuffed shirts.

"He calls himself the Friendly Psychiatrist. He lies down on the couch with you. They call this socialized medicine."

"The greatest obstacle to the advancement of medicine is atrophy of the ear."

9. **Invent topicals:** A humorous reference to some topic or issue of the day-headline news.

President Ford: "I'm America's first instant president. The band is so confused, it doesn't know whether to play Hail to the Chief or You've Come a Long Way, Baby."

10. **Humorous definitions:**

"Adolescence is that period in a child's life when his parents become more difficult."

"Area of expertise means you do everything else worse."

"Statistics are like a bikini! What they reveal is interesting. What they conceal is vital!"

11. **Use "sight" laughs** with gimmicks.

"The Chairman has asked me to say a few words" (Lifts a sheaf of papers three inches thick).

A sheet of paper attached to a new set of By-Laws reads: SEX. Now that I have your attention . . . please discard the old and read the new set of By-Laws.

12. **Deliberate mispronunciations, puns, use of abbreviations, acronyms:** Adds a brief but sudden jolt in a formal lecture or discussion, or conversation.

"You're putting the emphasis on the wrong syl-la'ble."

"That's a SWAG" (Scientific wild-assed guess).

Bill Cosby in TV show, "Feeling Good," is a fertilized egg in a skit on prenatal care. He calls up to Mom to send down "some calcium and iron." When it clangs down, he responds with, "Thanks, that's real womb service."

Now that you are hooked on humor, there are a few precautions and warnings. In your enthusiasm, don't try to be "too darned funny" or pile on too many jokes, says Bob Orben (1972). Don't strain to add humor which doesn't fit the situation. Restraint is the keynote. Humor has a tendency, like anything else, to be destroyed by overuse. A few well-placed, well-timed funnies are much more effective. If you are giving a speech or a lecture, make your first story or joke a blockbuster. Everything after that will be funny. At least you will keep your audience awake waiting for the next one!

Never, never, tell a story or joke unless you like it yourself and really think it is funny. Not so funny that you are rolling in the aisles yourself. That will turn your audience off rather than on. But, because you enjoy it, you can give it the right tone. Practice it!

When you tell a story, pause afterwards. Give your audience a chance to "get it."

Above all, "think funny." Look for chances to use humor, collect materials and practice! Analyze the humor you use. If it falls flat, why did it? Try again. Don't get discouraged and don't expect perfect results. Being humorous five percent of the time is better than not being humorous at all. Once you try it, you may find you like it.

Humor is addictive!

# INCREASING YOUR HUMOROUS PERSPECTIVE

In addition to analyzing your current sense of humor, and understanding the techniques of comedy and comedy styles, there are a number of other suggestions, exercises and activities for adding more humor to your life and expanding your humorous attitude. As Steve Allen (1987) has said, begin to see and enjoy the humor in life around you in developing your sense of humor; make a habit of listening to comedy albums, seeing comedy films, works of gifted humorists. He believes it is possible to say something funny or at least have a funny thought about almost everything.

Opening yourself up to humor, looking for absurdities in life, and becoming more "playful" and less serious about life is the broad perspective. Activities and exercises for increasing our playfulness in a non-competitive way were developed by Weinstein and Goodman (1980). They created a new type of play that lets people be supportive and cooperative and open with each other, especially people "who need to defrost their refrigerators" and for people who would like to make situations they are in more playful (p. 7).

Carl Simonton, oncologist (1978), learned and taught his patients to juggle, and Steve Allen, Jr., a physician who uses humor to heal in programs he runs on stress reduction and sexuality, teaches his audience to juggle silk scarves or tennis balls. He says, "It's a way to give people permission to play and laugh and be silly in public and it's a metaphor for . . . learning things you thought were impossible" (Allen, 1987, p. 8).

Joel Goodman (1983) (The Humor Project), teaches the development of humor, learning skills, and practical uses for integrating humor into one's work and lifestyle. He suggests putting on your "candid camera" glasses and looking for humor, "discovering the ELF in yoursELF," to "get with a laughing with rather than a laughing at" and follow the Rule of the "5 Ps" . . . practice, practice, practice, practice, practice."

In summary, there are some practical suggestions to open yourself up to humor and to begin to incorporate humor into your life:

Seek out humor! Collect things that make you laugh and share them — cartoons, books, articles, cassettes, videotapes, jokes, funny sayings, humorous incidents or stories, memos, comic strips, funny props and gadgets, silly books and games. Set up a bulletin board or refrigerator with humorous items. Compose a "Ha-Ha Book." Fantasize using humor! How can you handle a stressful, difficult situation with humor? What could you have said, after an embarrassing moment? Save it up for the next time! Add humor to your family life, to your work, to all your relationships. Start family mealtimes or group meetings with a joke. Take a "humor break." Laugh every day! Learn to laugh at yourself! Keep a log of personal anecdotes! Exaggerate! Poke fun at yourself! Schedule more play in your life. Be silly! Can't remember a joke? Write it down. Tell it to someone three times and you've got it! And practice, practice.

Look for humor and it will find you!

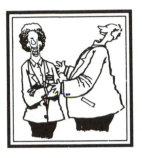

# 16
# Utilizing Humor: Some Beginning Guidelines

*"The time has come," the Walrus said, "To talk of many things: of shoes — and ships — and sealing-wax — of cabbages — and kings —and why the sea is boiling hot — and whether pigs have wings."*

Lewis Carroll,
Through the Looking Glass

Indeed, the time has come, Not to talk of cabbages and kings, but to speak to the heart of the matter for which this book was conceived. We have consistently affirmed that humor is one of the most valuable tools a health professional can have. We have spoken to the why; we have spoken to the what and the where of humor. We have begun to speak of the hows, and now we are down to the last how. How do we apply this knowledge, this new ability to be witty and humorous? How do we use this humor to improve communication, facilitate teaching, and help our patients intervene in the stresses and the anxieties with which they must cope? This is the heart of the matter. If we could call upon the Gryphon's "Classical master, who taught Laughing and Grief," all our problems would be solved.

There are three major groups with whom we as professionals communicate: our colleagues, our students, and our patients. We tend to stereotype our roles with each of these groups, as friend, teacher, and health-care giver. It follows that we tend also to stereotype our functional utilization of humor for each of these as meeting sociological needs, educational needs, and psychological needs, respectively. This may be the foremost function of humor in each of these roles. However, in our usual communication patterns we find this is not always so clear-cut. Meeting sociological needs with our friends and colleagues, we sometimes meet their psychological and educational needs as well. With our students we are sometimes social, and many times give psychological support. The same holds true with patients or clients. Our responses may be more in the direction of health teaching, and sometimes our communication is at a purely social level with no psychological overtones or directions. Guidelines for utilizing humor cut across roles and, just as there is no content area which is not subject to humor, so there is no one discrete function for the use of humor within various categories of persons. Rather, it is the time and situation which are the determining factors. For convenience, however, in presenting the recommendations for the practice of humor, the three broad sections of the communication framework, teaching, and intervention have been developed. The overlaps will be obvious, but the need to operationalize these interactions for specificity is also indicated.

# THE COMMUNICATION FRAMEWORK

Humor, we have said, is an indirect form of communication. Within health settings, it is apart from the "official normative system," and the choice to use humor is an optional matter. Because of the serious business of the hospital setting, Emerson expected to find in her study clearly defined areas and relationships where humor would or would not be used. She found instead that humor is permissible in almost any circumstances. This broad area includes colleagues, other staff, students, and patients. In only three instances did she find that humor did not occur: when patients were seriously threatening not to cooperate with staff; when the patient was extremely upset emotionally, and when the staff was interacting with the relatives or visitors of dying patients.

This freedom in the use of humor in actuality extends far beyond the hospital confines to other health agencies, to public health settings, to the home, to the classroom, and to society in general. However, within this freedom, if a choice to use humor is made, there are some informal social rules, and conventions or understandings about the initiation and conduct of humorous communication which must be considered.

Emerson (1963) has succinctly summarized the circumstances under which the choice to use humor in preference to other forms of indirect communication is made:

> a) A humorous tone is appropriate in the situation. b) It is possible to introduce a playful note without disrupting the serious business. c) There is relatively more consensus and intimacy among the participants (as indicated, for example, by similarity in age, sex, and position in the organization) so that the chance of a misunderstanding about whether humor is intended is reduced. d) The actor is willing to take the risk that the message will be ignored. e) A relatively high degree of exemption from responsibility is desired. f) The actor has the social role of fool, or is personally expected to joke (p. 47-48).

In making a choice to use humor, the initiator must also assess the receptivity of the other or others to his humor. Certain cues may indicate this acceptance: a previous joking relationship; ongoing humorous interaction; past or present initiations of humor by the other person; a feeling tone of receptivity as indicated by smiling, twinkling eyes, etc.; or a feeling of warmth, empathy and trust.

The initiator must also know his audience. He must evaluate whether the content will be understood, that the content will not be offensive, and that the message conveyed by the humor will be acceptable.

Once the decision to use humor is made, if it is to be successful, a framework must be established which is recognized by all concerned. The joke-frame says in effect: This is a joke. It is in fun. It is not serious. This joke-frame, says William Fry (1963), is similar to a play-frame and is as vital to situation jokes as it is to canned or formal jokes or practical jokes (p. 161). The establishment of this joke-frame involves two basic rules or components:

The first rule is that the initiator must make it very clear that he is joking and that humor is his intent, particularly when it is initiated in a nonhumorous setting. The cues that humor is being initiated may be verbal or nonverbal. Verbal cues are actual statements such as "Let me tell you a story," "Have you heard this one?" "This'll kill 'ya." Most cues, however, are in the form of nonverbal metacommunications. They signal that there is a change in the interaction. The signal may be a gesture, a shift in posture, a change in facial expression or tone of voice. The person may smile, wink, or get a "twinkle in his eyes." His face may "light up." The tone of his voice may become lighter, teasing, or flippant. He may chuckle or giggle.

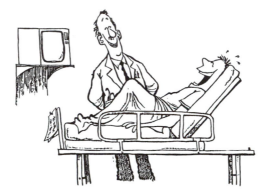

Sometimes, a dead-pan style of delivery, which is in direct contrast to these cues, may be used. In that context, the delivery is a joke in itself. It is generally used only when the relationship between the participants is such that it will be understood. That is, either this has occurred before in the relationship, or the content of the humor is so obvious and so outrageous that it can only be assumed to be humorous. A sudden shift to dialect or to mispronounced words or distorted phrases or an obvious misinterpretation of a situation are examples of content which are enhanced by the dead-pan delivery.

The second rule in the joking framework is that the recipient of the joke must acknowledge the humor, unless he chooses to imply that the humor is inappropriate, at which time the joke-frame is dissolved and the humor is lost. A lack of response may also mean that the recipient did not understand the humor or failed to "get the joke." In the case of a patient who is lethargic or in pain, he may understand, perhaps even appreciate, the humor, but physically may be unable to respond. In either case, the joke-frame will not be set. The "license to joke" given by the recipient is usually acknowledged by a laugh or a smile. Sometimes, it may be a groan! A verbal response like, "You're funny, man!" or "That's a good one!" may occur. A counter-joke or humorous remark by the recipient may set up a continued banter or humorous exchange. Once a joke-frame is thus set or established, future encounters or joking relationships are likely to occur.

The general communication framework for humor is applicable in any situation whether it be a one-to-one relationship or a group relationship, between staff and patient, between student and teacher, between colleagues or in setting the tone of a ward, a clinic, a classroom, or a professional conference. We will speak specifically to patient-staff interaction and to student-teacher interaction in the next sections, so an example from the same national nursing conference referred to previously might clarify this communication framework.

At a general session on the third morning of the conference, during a panel discussion, one of the panelists, representing a federal government agency, was speaking on the availability of federal funds to do what was needed in continuing education in nursing. She asked the audience to react spontaneously to what they saw as the future goals in continuing education and some of the needs to meet these goals. Several of the young leaders spoke to the lack of avenues for the preparation of identified potential leaders. Rather than a positive acknowledgment and acceptance of these individuals' personal ambitions and goals to be leaders, a condemnation of "smart-mouths" like themselves was often encountered. Getting to be a leader almost required a subtle denial of such ambition. As a result, the persons sometimes had the competency and sometimes not when they "fell into" the positions of leadership. Actual apprenticeships and internships with experts like the panelist was the solution these young persons from the audience were proposing.

The panelist acknowledged the need for leaders and the need for legitimized avenues of preparation and then said, "but let me tell you a mythological story."

> There is a $10,000 bill in the center of a conference table. At one corner of this table is sitting an Expert Administrator, at another corner is the Easter Bunny, at another corner is Santa Claus, and at the fourth corner is a Bumbling Administrator. Only one of the four can have the money. At the sound of the gong, who do you think got the $10,000 bill?
>
> The answer is: The Bumbling Administrator, of course, because all the others are mythological figures!

There were many messages conveyed: Don't put us on a pedestal. We're not perfect. Don't you expect to be perfect. There are no absolute experts. What makes one leader effective may be ineffective if tried by others.

The humor used was very successful in this instance because the framework for communication through humor had been established. There had been many cues throughout that morning that humor was acceptable because both speakers and audience had made witty comments and there had been much laughter. The one young leader's reference to herself as a "smart-mouth," which got a big laugh, as well as other witty remarks, communicated to the panelist that she could also respond with humor. She also knew her audience and knew they were specific-centered enough to get the message conveyed by the joke without needing a serious lecture which would have been inappropriate at the time. Her self-depreciating joke also brought the tone of the meeting from a confrontation of "What have you not done for us and what are you going to do about it?" back to the original sharing, congenial atmosphere of what are we going to do about it.

# PATIENT INTERVENTION

The humor used in the situation just described was very effective because the panelist had assessed the situation, knew her audience, and recognized that a humorous intervention would be appropriate. There was a subsequent reduction in tension and a return to social interaction. She probably did not think through the process for her choice, but if she had, what might that process be? How can we, as practitioners of health care, apply that same process to assisting our patients and families to cope with the tensions and stresses they encounter? As helping professionals we expect our intervention choices to be based on some sound rationale.

The framework for this process is actually no different from the problem-solving process employed in many other situations and in any other intervention technique: making an assessment through collection of data; identifying the problem; determining the mode of intervention, and then evaluating the results. The difference is that, in this instance, the base is the knowledge and information we have gathered about the concept of humor. We must recognize also that this process has rarely been applied in any systematic way to the use of humor. When humor has been used, more often than not, it has been a spontaneous, intuitive activity rather than a planned one.

It is true that at the present time situational or spontaneous humor is the most common form of humor seen in the health setting. But this may be because humor has not been thought of in any other way. However, by enough conscious, deliberate use of humor, we can make the most out of situational humor which occurs, and become skilled enough to begin to be spontaneous and create our own situational humor without always having a preconceived plan. As with any other interpersonal and intervention skill, we integrate the theoretical and problem-solving base into our action, so that the process becomes one that we initiate "almost without thinking." "Practicing" humor has its drawbacks, since if humor seems "practiced" it destroys the humor. However, this is the initial risk we must take if we are ever to become skilled. It is like our first attempts at giving injections or interviewing. We are awkward and hesitant. Yet this is the learning process which is universally accepted.

The first step in the process is assessment, or know your audience. Who is your patient? What is his culture? His age? His personality? What is his sense of humor? What cues can you pick up that he has been using humor as a mechanism for coping? Does he tease and laugh and smile? Does he initiate humor? Make jokes? What are the cues that he would be receptive to your humorous attempts? Have you established the kind of basic relationship of trust and empathy which says to him, "I understand, I'm here to help you. But things aren't so bad. Can't we laugh about it?"

Including a "humor history" in our initial patient assessment would give us a practical way of assessing the individuals's response to humor. Moody (1978) has used a set of questions in his practice such as: What role did humor play in the person's family in growing up? Was he teased as a child? What kinds of jokes or humor does he like best? What is his favorite joke? How often does he laugh (p. 119)? Herth (1984) in her assessment which she calls her "Funny Bone History" adds: What kinds of things make you laugh? How do you feel when you laugh? When was the last time you played? Do you find humor a source of relaxation? She then asks her clients to write down for the next week each time they laughed and what made them laugh.

We must also assess the client's receptivity to the humor. What are the indications he might not be receptive? Is he very serious? Is he negative to humor or to certain styles of humor? Be sensitive to his humor preference. Be aware of his education level. Can he get the point of your humor? Consider the age of the client. What will be funny to a teenager may not be funny or understood by the elderly.

Is he emotionally too distraught and too anxious or too angry? Assess his level of anxiety. If it is too high, we know that his decreased ability to concentrate, to listen, to focus may obviate any attempt at humor. Humor might even be irritating or be taken as a negation of his perception of the seriousness of the situation.

We must also assess the patient's physiological condition. Is he is pain? Are drugs clouding his consciousness? Is he confused? Is he facing organic changes? The patient may not be able to respond to humor. Back-stage humor, or humor around the patient but not including him, can be, at this time, irritating and annoying to the patient. However, a patient who may not be able to communicate may still be receptive.

> An elderly gentleman who had had a stroke was unable to talk but was still alert. The student nurse carried on a one-sided conversation with him as she bathed and cared for him each day. Knowing that he, too, lived on a tobacco farm, she reminisced about her childhood and growing up on the farm, and her secret trips behind the barn to learn to smoke and chew and spit tobacco like her father! The patient burst out laughing! It was his first physical response. The next day when the nurse returned, he gave her a big smile and said "tobacco!" — his first word in his subsequent recovery!

The second step is to determine the problem or the need for

which humor might be the choice for intervention. If the patient jokes or uses humor himself, what need is he trying to meet? Evaluate the content of the humor and the situation in which it is occurring. Does it seem to be effective for him in coping with that stress or that need? How have others, including yourself, responded to his humor? Have you encouraged it by laughing and smiling in return and showing your acceptance? Not laughing, but responding negatively or with seriousness to a patient's humor, should be looked at carefully. Do we insult him or destroy our communication with him because he feels reprimanded?

Once we have made our basic assessment and identified the need or a problem area, we can then determine how, what kind, and when we should initiate the humor, and establish the joke-frame for using it. The humor itself should be based on the professional's own style, the situation, the content and the need, utilizing all the techniques described previously. It may be a witticism, a teasing remark, a joke, or even a funny anecdote that may have happened to another patient in the same circumstance or with the same anxiety.

> A medical technician who has come to draw blood for a laboratory test responds to the very anxious patient's "Will this hurt?" with exaggerated antics and "It will be the worst pain in your life!" And she laughs!

> A patient listening to the therapist explaining the loss of hair as one of the side effects of the chemotherapy, grinned and said, "Well, I guess Yul Brenner will just have to be the second sexiest bald-headed man!" The therapist often relates this anecdote when she is educating other patients.

Once the humorous interaction has occurred, evaluate it. Was it effective? Was the need met? Was the tension reduced? The message conveyed? If so, further intervention may be unnecessary or even inappropriate. One of the functions of humor, as we have repeatedly stated, is to provide a mechanism for dealing with issues and transmitting messages which might be unacceptable if stated directly.

However, rather than getting a laugh, did your humor fall flat? Or did it get a negative response? If it was unsuccessful, analyze why. Was it your technique, was it the humorous content, or was the patient not ready to accept the message? Not many unsuccessful jokes occur, but when they do it may be that "some implicit message not suitable for direct communication is stripped of its camouflage." If the patient responds within a serious frame, failure is implied. It may be that he is reacting to the content of the humor. A slightly risque joke may be acceptable; a vulgar one may not. Political, racial, ethnic, or religious jokes may offend. Or somehow the humor failed because the initiator missed some cue or failed to carry out his performance well. It might be helpful to say at that point, to the patient, "My joke didn't go over very well. I wonder why?"

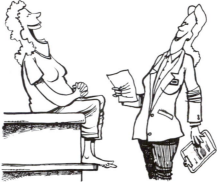

We might look at two examples of attempts at a practical joke, one of which succeeded and the other failed.

> A patient who had been hospitalized for a long period of time in complete balanced traction was scheduled for further surgery. All of the staff had excellent rapport with the patient. They filled a 5 cc syringe with orange juice, and most of the staff went into the room to help "give" the "preoperative" injection. The staff reported there was a general good feeling by both patient and staff and an evidenced relief of anxiety on the part of the patient.

> In another instance, following a hemorrhoidectomy, an enema was ordered for a young male patient; the nurse, who felt she had a good relationship with the patient, thought she would tease him, and brought into the room a huge milk bucket and the largest hose she could find. The patient took one look, ran to the bathroom and refused to come out, unable to see the joke.

In both attempts at humor, the staff felt they had established a good relationship with the patient, yet one failed and the other succeeded. We might wonder if the nurse in the second situation failed to cue the patient that it was a joke! Certainly the pain and embarrassment are more intense with a hemorrhoidectomy than with a preoperative hypodermic, so that the content of the humor was a "touchy" one which the nurse may not have appropriately assessed. There may be other factors contributing to the success or failure which the individuals in the situation could identify if they pursued such an analysis.

Although most humor, as an indirect communication, may serve its purpose without further intervention, humor may also be used as a vehicle for opening up a serious discussion. "A joke may serve as a trial balloon to invite a discussion of doubtful propriety" (Emerson, 1969, p. 172). The negotiations to suspend the general guidelines for joking may be initiated by either party, patient or staff. The health professional and patient may banter back and forth to determine if the other is willing to open a discussion. The more the joker acknowledges that his humor may have a serious import, the easier it is to transpose the humor to a serious discussion. On the other hand, if the patient is not ready to face the taboo topic, he can deny the seriousness and end the negotiation, at which point the staff person should not pursue the topic, but return to the humor facade or terminate the interaction. Such denial indicates to the professional that the patient's use of humor was a face-saving device. In the emotion-laden areas of death and dying the patient or staff "backing-off" from joking about dying is very common. On the other hand, humor may also be used as a means for opening up and allowing the patient to discuss his fears and his concerns.

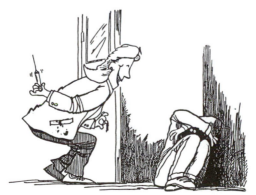

Humor may also be used as a pattern of communication in a long-term relationship to facilitate the therapeutic process. A graduate student in psychiatric nursing, working with a young black woman whose acute psychotic episode had been precipitated by her mother's death found that humor became a way of reaching her. The patient's mother had treated her as a retarded child, so that she felt oppressed and controlled, lacked confidence in herself, and was angry at having been thrust in that role. The humorous exchanges and the nurse's use of self-depreciating humor was an attempt to have the patient see her as a friend rather than another controlling mother. For example, when the patient said, she "made spaghetti for dinner last night. It was just canned spaghetti. I'm a can cook," the nurse responded with "You're not alone!" and they both laughed. By the time they were terminating, the patient was calling her "a friend in a professional way" because "a friend knows what you can do."

This same nurse utilized the humor that occurred within a therapy group and picked up on it as a way to integrate the group and relieve tension.

> In one session the patients were talking about how irritating it was when some patients wore soiled clothing and did not bathe. One patient who often used humor, said, "Well, my bath days are Monday and Thursday, but it seems like I never take them on those days. I had one in January . . ." And as the group started to laugh, the nurse said, "Whether you needed it or not, right, Jack?" At which point another patient quipped, "It was a New Year's resolution!"

The value of the comic effect and humor as a way to control dysfunctional behavior in outer space was suggested early in the space flight programs (Friedman, 1963). The fear, the unknown dangers, the isolation, sensory deprivation, boredom, and loss of social contact were some of the socio-psychological stresses identified. Investigators hypothesized that comic laughter could be a means for prevention and amelioration of these reactions. The suggested activities were to provide audiovisual media and tapes of comedy shows, cartoons, classic stories, etc.

However, as the space program progressed, it became evident that the astronauts and staff had incorporated humor into their way of life. Those who followed the space flights and the interchanges between space crew and ground crew heard many quips, little jokes, and humorous comments. When the first ship to reach the moon was taking off to return to the command module, the unexpected strains of "Here We Go, Into the Wild Blue Yonder," delighted the whole world.

Werner Von Braun in his many talks on "Exploration in Space" used humor to lighten this awesome subject and convey to the audience that it was "just a job." The astronauts often referred to the escape button which detached their compartment during launching in the event of danger as "the chicken switch" and boarding the ship as "walking the plank."

Always the key to the therapeutic and appropriate use of humor is being sensitive to whose needs are being met. There is a right time, a right place, a right style and the right content. It is always offered in the context of love, warmth, understanding and support, and is a laughing with and not a laughing at! Sarcasm, ridicule and ethnic put-down humor are non-therapeutic. Be sensitive to that fine line. Gallows humor is therapeutic for staff but may not be for the patient or family. Include the patient in the humor around him. Backstage humor or humor between staff that ignores the patient can be non-therapeutic. Constant clowning or joking may also become ineffective. Be sensitive to the time or place when humor is not the appropriate choice, when the patient may need to cry, be alone or need another intervention. Planned well, the use of humor can be as healing and therapeutic for the individual as is the spontaneous situational humor which occurs in the health care setting.

# APPLICATION OF HUMOR TO THE CLIMATE OF HEALTH CARE

In addition to the use of humor with the individual, humor can also be added to the climate of the health care setting. An atmosphere, a team effort and the use of a variety of humorous materials and activities can enhance the use of humor as a therapeutic tool.

The use of humor as a planned team effort, observed in the initial research (Robinson, 1978), was effective in the recovery of elderly widow who had become depressed following major surgery. Each of the staff used joking, teasing, and humor as part of the plan of care. Humor, however, was used extensively as a form of communication by the nursing team on this unit and set the tone for the patients to express their feelings in this way. The head nurse also used humor, joking and teasing with her patients as she made rounds. This seemed to be the most comfortable way for her to communicate. Through humor, she was able to ascertain patients' needs, giving them the feeling she was concerned about them, but reassuring them that their being in the hospital was not so deadly serious an event.

The nursing team members also used humor to relieve their own anxieties and stresses. Besides the usual bantering and teasing, the blackboard in the locker room next to the nurse's station became a daily source of humor with the graduates, student nurses, and aides all contributing cartoons. One chalk drawing showed bedraggled, weary students on night duty with the dates of their service crossed off each morning and the instructor with wings and a jumpsuit hovering above. Another was of a student on "Preops" struggling with a syringe twice as big as herself with patients running in all directions and the student saying, "But it's only 1 cc. of each."

In summary, the use of humor on this ward was a therapeutic force. It created a warm climate and promoted good staff interpersonal relationships. The warmth was transmitted to the patients who, in turn, were able to use humor as a method of relieving the stresses of hospitalization. Yet the use of humor was controlled: the realistic needs of patients were not lost in the laughter, and the humor could be turned off when it was not effective.

Norman Cousins' reported use of humorous materials (Candid Camera videotapes, films of the Marx Brothers, humorous books) to stimulate his healing laughter (1979) was a stimulus for the development of "humor rooms" and the integration of other humorous props and activities.

The first of the "Humor Rooms" was developed by St. Joseph Hospital in Houston, Texas, for their cancer unit. Their "living room" is a bright, warm, cheery place where patients, families and staff can gather and share humor and "living." It is filled with humorous materials, books, videos, films, cassettes, Ha-Ha, scrapbooks of cartoons and humor, a piano and a TV. Parties and bingo are held, clowns and entertainers are invited in. The staff is encouraged to utilize humor as part of their care. Inspired by this, other humor rooms for Oncology patients have sprung up. DeKalb General Hospital in Decatur, Georgia, called their room "The Lively Room," (after a Mr. Lively who donated the initial funds).

Across the country, Veterans Hospitals, rehabilitation hospitals, nursing homes, childrens units and other general hospitals have incorporated rooms or other humorous activities. "Laff carts" containing humorous materials and props are circulated from room to room for non-ambulatory patients; there is closed circuit TV with comedy stations and patient education materials; "clown rounds" by staff, and posters, cartoons, bulletin boards and white newsprint on the wall for patients to add their creations. One gynecology clinic has added cartoons to the ceiling of their examining rooms! Another clinic for chronically ill patients asks them to prepare "Joy Bags" filled with things that bring joy and make them laugh, for the "rough times" (Herth, 1984). Geriatric centers have jokes and humor sharing sessions. Mason jars filled with printed jokes and cartoons are passed out to patients with their medications. A variety of props are used: teddy bears dangling from bed frames, puppets, other "huggables," balloons, bubble pipes and other mirth inducing materials which convey the feeling of life and wellness.

# HUMOR IN HEALTH EDUCATION

The use of humor in patient/client education is a positive tool. A little story, cartoon or joking sets the stage for decreasing the anxiety and increasing the receptivity to learning, to listening and hearing the facts about the serious subject, whether it is diabetes, heart surgery, AIDS, medications, or how to manuever with a cast! Humorous written materials have been developed which can be shared, like *The Sensuous Heart: Guidelines for Sex After a Heart Attack* (Cambre, 1978).

> One anesthesiologist has a stock answer to the usual question asked by pre-surgical patients, "How much will the anesthesia cost?" "Oh, about $100. $1 to go to sleep and $99 for waking up! Most patients buy the whole package."

Health education for health promotion, through the use of humor, play and laughter, has increased in popularity. There are courses, workshops, conferences and programs for the public in general, and for specific groups and professionals, to improve our lifestyles, for dealing with the stresses of living and for learning how to broaden one's humor perspective. Health promotion books have been published: *The Laughter Prescription*: How to achieve health, happiness, and peace of mind through humor (Peter & Dana, 1982); *The Smile Connection*: How to use humor in dealing with people (Blumenfeld & Alpern, 1986); *A Laughing Place*: The art and psychology of positive humor in love and adversity (Hegeseth III, 1988); and *The Healing Power of Humor*: Techniques for getting through loss, setbacks, upsets, disappointments, difficulties, trials, tribulations and all that not-so-funny stuff (Klein, 1989). All are excellent sources for teaching how and why and when to incorporate humor in our lives for our good health.

# TEACHING HUMOR

Since humor has not been a concept which traditionally has been included in the education of the health professional and there are no present guidelines, how can we begin to teach the practice of humor as a therapeutic tool in the helping process? What learning experiences to utilize humor can we develop for use in the classroom, whether that classroom be part of a basic program, a graduate program, or a continuing education program?

In the chapter "Humor in Education," we outlined four areas for the educator to consider. The first two — utilizing humor as a catalyst in the learning process itself, and, facilitating the process of socialization into the health professions — have been discussed. The last two — teaching the concepts and the practice of humor, and modeling the use of humor as a vehicle for facilitating the other three — will be the focus of this section.

The beginning steps for the educator to incorporate humor into the teaching-learning process were outlined in the chapters "Developing a Sense of Humor" and "The Techniques of Comedy." Looking at ourselves, assessing our own attitudes and style of humor, and then cultivating the basic techniques in creating humor are as vital to our teaching posture as it is to our practice with patients. Modeling the use of humor in the classroom and establishing that kind of relationship provides the vehicle for the student to feel comfortable in relating in this way with patients and colleagues.

In addition to creating personal humor, the teacher, of course, has access to many other humorous articles, cartoons, poems, quotations, posters, and jokes which can be introduced into the class presentation to emphasize a concept or issue or to initiate a discussion.

A small pre-test (1975) was conducted of the materials presented in the chapters "Humor in Education" and "The Techniques of Comedy" on creating humor in the classroom. Twenty-one instructors were asked to read this "Guide for Incorporating Humor in the Teaching-Learning Process," react to it, and then attempt to use the guide to either add humor to their teaching strategies or to analyze the humor they felt they were already using. They were asked to keep a log for one month, evaluate the usefulness of the Guide, and then ask their students to evaluate their performance. The students were not to be told that the study was being conducted until completion.

Most of the instructors only reacted to the Guide and did not test it, due to pressures of time or not being involved in enough actual classroom teaching during the period of the study. Several frankly stated they had doubts about their ability to do this; others felt the Guide was too "cook-bookish" and were uncomfortable with formal jokes. Others, who were already considered "funny" instructors by their peers, suggested that this author review the tapes of their lectures (some of which had been done prior to the study). Twenty of these tapes were subsequently analyzed. Several of the instructors also wrote up material which they had used in their classes. Only two of the group actually tested the Guide and had their students evaluate them.

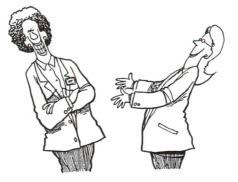

One of these two faculty members honestly felt that she had no sense of humor and was not a "joke-telling" person, but made a deliberate effort to utilize the guidelines. She attempted to be more "light-hearted" and simply "to keep the old Irish maxim, you may as well laugh grief as cry it." She made more frequent attempts to laugh over minor errors and felt, thus, she was less threatening to the students. She utilized a slide-cartoon series called "The Long Ranger" in a class on Perspective Medicine, discussing long-range planning for health care and health hazard appraisal. The series is a take-off on the Lone Ranger; she introduced the audiovisual aid with a comment that this was to be enjoyed and students should not try to take notes.

Interestingly enough, the students' evaluations of her ranged from not noticing any change to yes, there was one. One student noticed the instructor was "very cheerful, but thought it was spring fever." Moreover, despite the instructor's perception of herself as "not humorous," two of the students felt there was nothing unusual because this instructor was always in good humor, ready to tell a joke or laugh at another joke or funny situation, and didn't see how she could become more humorous "without being ridiculous."

The other instructor who utilized the Guide and had her students evaluate her was one whom everyone felt was absolutely the funniest instructor around. Yet the instructor said, "They laugh, but I don't know why they do." In this instance, she asked another instructor to observe her in class and record those instances in which laughter occurred. In addition, this author reviewed the tapes of her lectures. The analysis showed that her humor consisted primarily of very spontaneous, situational witticisms which came out in such a dry, droll fashion that the delivery was as important to the humorous communication as the content itself. The content is typical of situational humor that taken out of context may not be funny at all. One needs to be involved in the situation to get the full impact of the amusement. One student commented that the instructor had a mischievous twinkle in her eye that suggested "chronic humor." Are these cues to the attitude about which we have been talking?

She very often mispronounced words, like "eveel" for evil and "royal" for rural and then added as the students laughed, "I hear you! I should take a course in diction."

Other examples:

> When the class asked her "to slow down" in her lecturing, she responded with ". . . slow down? Sorry, I did say we'd mosey on through the respiratory unit, didn't I?"

> In attempting to draw on the blackboard a sketch of the pedicle of the kidney, with which she was having difficulty, she said, "I can't wait till we get to kidneys. I can draw those!"

> In describing how to count seconds, she said one should say to oneself, ". . . 1001, 1002, 1003 . . . . Is that right?"

> In talking about loss of time sense in a particular disease, she said "Time sure flies when you're having fun."

> She used herself in many situations, e.g., describing her own habit of smoking when talking about emphysema.

Fifty-six of her 100 students evaluated her; again, the comments ranged from very positive statements about her humor to one who did not notice anything funny. Does this verify the fact that humor is a matter of individual perception and receptivity?

The students were asked if the humor improved the class and increased learning. The responses were generally positive. It made the class "less dull," "provided a relaxed atmosphere more conducive to learning," and made the instructor "seem more human." "One seems to remember facts when they are associated with something funny and interesting." Humor "revived lagging attention," "Kept me awake," and "alleviated the anxiety associated with learning," students noted.

An analysis of the humor from the 20 tapes plus the written descriptions of humor used could be broken down into three major categories:
1. sponteneous, situational humor;
2. canned variety;
3. reference to humor or use of humor; and two sub-categories: those that:
   1. related to the topic or subject of the lecture; or
   2. were extraneous to the subject matter.

In listening to the lecture, there were many times that laughter occurred which must have related to a gesture, facial expression, or some other nonverbal cues which the listener could not see and therefore, could not ascertain the reason for the laughter.

Most of the incidents of humor were of the spontaneous situational type. Many of them were simple pleasantries. They were about equally divided between those directly related to the subject and those external to the topic. A directly related example of humor occurred during a panel discussion on kidney transplants.

> One of the students asked if patients who needed transplants wait anxiously for donors. One of the head nurses on the panel

responded. "I asked my patients if they lay awake on Memorial Day weekend listening for screeching brakes and they only laughed. Of course there is a shortage of donors since the speed limit was set at 55!"

Humor external to the subject area was an aside: "Is it hot in here or am I going through menopause?" And then followed some quips about age and Premarin ads.

Humor of the canned variety consisted of those already prepared jokes, cartoons, poems, etc. During a class on obesity, the instructor used several of these. She gave some definitions of fad diets: "A rhythm method of girth control" or "A grim cycle of lose-a-little, gain a little more." She opened the class with this poem on a transparency.

> Fading is the taper waist,
> Shapeless grows the shapely limb,
> And although severely laced,
> Spreading is the figure trim,
> Stouter than I used to be,
> Still more corpulent grow I.
> There will be too much of me
> In the coming bye and bye.
>
> Gilbert and Sullivan

There were two references to humor itself. The "funny" instructor several times said, "Write all those jokes down, I'll use them again next year." Another instructor, in discussing crisis intervention, was relating her own crisis when her gynecologist during an examination asked, "When did you notice the lump in your breast?" She said to the class, "I responded by making a joke. That's my coping mechanism. But he didn't laugh, which said to me, it is serious. Instead he asked if I had a choice of a surgeon."

This study is only a beginning in analyzing humor in the classroom and evaluating methods for learning to model it. The feedback regarding the guidelines themselves were helpful. The one major accomplishment of the study was the change in attitude regarding the cultivation of humor expressed by many of the educators. As one educator, who initially admitted to feeling dubious about such a Guide based on "you either had it or didn't . . .", said:

Consciously thinking about humor is the first step rather than envying the person who is "naturally witty." I suppose we all have self-conscious fears of coming across poorly and using humor alien to our style. Yet there is only one way to find out what one is comfortable with and can use effectively.

The other aspect educators must consider is how to teach the intervention skills to students. What kind of learning experiences can we provide once the basic theoretical content is given? There are several suggested methods which could be used.

To help students to look at their own styles and attitudes toward humor, they could be asked to write down and relate either a favorite joke or the funniest thing that ever happened to them. An analysis of the joke is also a way to evaluate their knowledge of the basic concept. This might be done as an individual assignment or a group activity.

Role-playing situations in the classroom in which humor is used might be another learning activity. This can be a demonstration by the instructor or an assignment to the students. Brief descriptions of patient situations in which some basic feeling such as tension, anxiety, anger, or embarrassment is evident can be developed. Utilizing these, the students make an assessment and then role-play how they would relieve these feelings through humor. In management classes at graduate and continuing education levels, role playing can help staff approach management about problems and issues, or help administrators approach staff in supervising, evaluating or making changes through the avenue of humor. Any of these may be a spontaneous classroom activity or an overnight assignment so that the student deliberately plans an intervention. Role-playing in the classroom helps to relieve anxiety and makes the anticipated situation in reality less awkward.

In a beginning class in nursing, two instructors demonstrated how humor can be used to reduce a patient's anxiety during preoperative care. First, the instructors played the role in a very negative way, with loud and raucous joking remarks to each other, asking the patient if she wanted her gallstones in a bottle so she could display them on her mantle at home. The "patient" obviously cringed and grimaced and huddled under the sheets. Then the scene was replayed in a positive fashion, using a joke to initiate a conversation about her fears. The "nurse" said, "You look as though you'd like to get out of bed and run. You remind me of a cartoon I saw. There is an operating room with six gowned and masked figures standing around an empty operating room table. The surgeon is looking around and saying, "Come, come, now, one of you must be the patient." The role-playing "patient" giggled and said, "Yeah, that's what I'd like to do, hide!" A discussion of her fears ensued.

The faculty role-playing or demonstrating some skill in a very negative way often is very humorous because of its absurdity and gets lots of laughs. This can be a means of saying, "All right, how would you do this appropriately?"

Instructors also being able to relate their own humorous experiences as students or staff help the students, who usually have unrealistic expectations for themselves, to relax and feel that they can laugh at their own mistakes if teachers can laugh at theirs. Making use of situation humor in the classroom also adds to the instructor's humanness. On one occasion the instructor, who was demonstrating how to move a patient in bed, first took her shoes off (high heels), next her glasses which had fallen down, and then remarked, "I promise you, that's the last thing I'll take off."

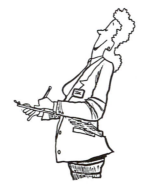

There may be a variety of other learning experiences which could be devised for "practicing" the use of humor. Of course, encouraging the student to add humor to assessment of patients in planning care in the clinical area provides the opportunity for the actual experience necessary to develop the skill in intervention.

One educational program in nursing has reported the use of humor in their program (Watson & Emerson, 1988). The concept is formally introduced in the second semester. In order to help students "think" humor, they are asked to keep a humor diary, share their favorite jokes and cartoons, and to caption a picture. In practice, the student wears a smile/frown button, which is turned up for good performance, and turned down when a "bummer" occurs. On holidays or special days (Halloween, St. Patrick's Day) students wear appropriate silly dress which patients also enjoy. And, they learn to discriminate between constructive and destructive humor and to begin to recognize situations in which it is appropriate to plan humor as an intervention.

There may be other health professional groups who are beginning to incorporate humor more formally into their educational programs and into their practices. We know that Norman Cousins, as adjunct professor at UCLA School of Medicine, has been involved in teaching medical students to communicate more effectively and is involved in a research project studying the biochemical properties of all the positive emotions. We need, as health professionals, to learn to use this powerful tool.

# SUMMARY

There are still many unanswered questions in this whole area of humor and much more research to be done. But, we need to begin. We need to explore the use of humor, to try out various approaches, to experiment.

The DK theory is what we operate on in most helping relationships anyway, says one authority. DK stands for degrees of knowledge, ranging from 'don't know' to 'damn confident!'

> The DK theory is very simply applied: To each and every professional action, the worker simply attaches a mental subscript, DK = _____%, referring to the percentage or proportion of ignorance actually operating in this particular action. One must act on the best available knowledge, to be sure, but one must be equally aware of the degree of knowledge involved in one's actions (Bloom, 1975).

So, let us have the courage to try. After all, jokes never really "killed" anyone!

# Conclusions

*The fun two human beings in sensitive communion can generate between them-selves is what it all comes down to. We make ourselves happy by making each other happy. And why not? We are all so capable to making each other miserable that the telling of jokes, or the communication of humor in general seems an indispensable balance in the seesaw of human relations.*

Mindess

Harvey Mindess has said it so well. Laughter is indispensable. This phenomenon of humor and laughter with which we as human beings have been endowed is more than just fun and trivia! It is a healthy, therapeutic tool that we must learn how to develop, to cultivate and to use in a more forceful way. It helps us to survive. It gives us a perspective on life and helps us to achieve that balance, that equilibrium that is healthy and healing.

The purpose of this book has been to pull together, as a beginning effort, the available knowledge in the area of humor and health. We have only scratched the surface. There is much more to be done.

The initial studies attempted for the development of this book were exploratory in nature. Further research is needed. Research in the area of intervention, in what makes humor successful and what factors cause it to fail, is of prime importance. Still needed are definitive studies on the use of humor in various cultures or ethnic groups related to health and illness. Also, sorely needed, is definitive research on the long term effects on health, on healing, and on longevity.

In conclusion, in my enthusiasm and strong belief in the value of humor, I may have projected a one-sided view: that humor is all. Perhaps you have already recognized that because humor has been so neglected, I have been rather adamant about its increased use. However, I feel impelled to remind the health professional that humor must always be placed in perspective to the whole, that whole a human being.

In the total plan for the care of our patient, humor is one communication tool, one mechanism for coping, one teaching methodology. It is useful and therapeutic in the right situation and the right time. As with anything else, a good thing can be overdone; a judicious amount is the right amount. If a drug is good, three times the dosage is not better. There will be times, as with grief when there is a need for lightness and humor, that humor will turn to tears, when laughter no longer suffices. What is important is to understand humor, to become skilled in recognizing when it is appropriate and beneficial, and to encourage its use, not ignore it.

In this age of rapid medical and technological advances, when the fears and threats of being replaced and controlled by machines are a reality, humor can be the means for retaining the humanness in the health professions. Humor is exclusively a human condition. Adlai Stevenson once paraphrased Socrates' famous statement, "The unexamined life is not worth living," with "Life without laughter is not worth examining."

# References

Adair, J.; Deuschle, K. W. (1970). *The people's health, medicine and anthropology in a Navajo community*. New York: Appleton-Century-Crofts.

Adams, J. (1968). *Encyclopedia of humor*. New York: Bobbs-Merrill.

Allen, S. (1981). *Funny people*. New York: Stein & Day.

Allen, S. (1982). *More funny people*. New York: Stein & Day.

Allen, S. (1986). A sense of humor: Steve Allen's own brand of laugh therapy. *Cope Magazine*. November, pp. 10-13.

Allen, S. with J. Wollman (1987). *How to be funny*. New York: McGraw-Hill.

Allport, G. W. (1961). *The individual and his religion*. New York: Macmillan.

Andrus Foundation (1983). *Humor: the tonic you can afford*. Los Angeles: University of Southern California.

Apte, M. L. (1985). *Humor and laughter: an anthropological approach*. Ithica, NY: Cornell University Press.

Armour, R. (1963). *The medical muse*. New York: McGraw Hill.

Armour, R. (1974). A short course in geriatric medicine. *Geriatrics*. January, pp. 125-129.

Averill, J. R. (1969). Automatic response patterns during sadness and mirth. *Psychophysiology*, 5, 399-414.

Baker, R. A. (1963). *Psychology in the wry*. Princeton, NY: Van Nostrand.

Baker, R. A. (1967). *A stress analysis of a strapless evening gown and other essays for a scientific age*. Englewood Cliffs, NJ: Prentice-Hall.

Bariaud, F. (1989). Age difference in children's humor. In P. E. McGhee (ed.) *Humor and children's development: A guide to practical applications* (pp. 15-45). New York: Haworth.

Bergler, E. (1956). *Laughter and the sense of humor*. New York: Intercontinental Medical Book Corp.

Bergson, H. (1900/1960). Laughter. In J. J. Enck, E. T. Forter & A. Whitley (eds.) *The comic in theory and practice* (pp.43- 64). New York: Appleton-Century-Crofts.

Berk, L. S.; Tan, S. A.; Fry, W. A.; Napier, B.; Lee, J. W.; Hubbard, R. W.; Lewis, J. E.; & Eby, W. C. (1989). Neuroendocrine and stress hormone changes during mirthful laughter. *The American Journal of the Medical Sciences*, *298*(6) pp. 390-396.

Berlyne, D. E. (1969). Laughter, humor and play. *Handbook of social psychology*, *3*, 795-813. Reading, MA: Addison-Wesley.

Bloch, S.; Browning, S.; & McGrath, G. (1983). Humor in group psychotherapy. *British Journal of Medical Psychology*, *56*, 89-97.

Bloch, S. (1987). Humor in Group Therapy. In W. F. Fry, Jr. & W. A. Salameh (eds.) *Handbook of Humor and Psychotherapy* (pp. 171-194). Sarasota, FL: Professional Resource Exchange.

Bloom, M. (1975). *The paradox of helping: Introduction to the philosophy of scientific practice.* New York: John Wiley and Sons.

Blumenfeld, E. & Alpern, L. (1986). *The smile connection.* Englewood Cliffs, NJ: Prentice-Hall.

Bornemeier, W. C. (1960). Sphincter-protecting hemorroidectomy. *American Journal of Proctocology*, *11*, 48-52.

Boskin, J. (1979). *Humor and social change in twentieth century America.* Boston: Trustees of the Public Library.

Bowen, E. S. [pseud] (1964). *Return to laughter.* Garden City, NY: The Natural History Library, Anchor Books, Doubleday.

Bradney, P. (1957). The joking relationship in industry. *Human Relations*, *14*, 170-187.

Brody, M. W. (1950). The meaning of laughter. *Psychoanalytic Quarterly*, *19*, 192-201.

Brown, J. (1958). *Perennially Yours, PROBIE.* New York: Springer Publishing.

Burma, J. H. (1946). Humor as a technique in race conflict. *American Sociological Review*, *11*, 710-715.

Bushnell, D. D. (1978). *The cathartic effect of laughter in comedy.* Unpublished doctoral dissertation. Santa Barbara: University of California.

Bushnell, D. D., Scheff, T. J. (1979). The cathartic effects of laughter on audiences. In H. Mindess & J. Turek (eds.), *The study of humor.* Los Angeles: Antioch University.

Collins, M. (1987). *Humor: An informal channel of communication used by institutionalized aged to express feelings of aggression due to personal deficits in power and status*. Unpublished doctoral dissertation. NY: Fairleigh Dickinson University.

Coombs, R. H., & Goldman, L. J. (1975). A situation of distressed arousal and strategies of emotional detachment, maintenance and discontinuity of coping mechanism in an intensive care unit. In L. Lofland (ed.) *Doing Social Life*. New York: Basic Books.

Coser, R. L. (1959). Some social functions of laughter. *Human Relations*, *12*, 171-182. And (1965). In J.K. Skipper & R.C. Leonard (Eds.), Social Interaction and Patient Care. Philadelphia: J.B. Lippincott.

Coser, R. L. (1960). Laughter among colleagues. *Psychiatry*, *23*, 81-95.

Cousins, N. (1979). *Anatomy of an illness*. New York: Norton.

Cousins, N. (1983). *The healing heart*. New York: Norton.

D'Antonio, I. J. (1989). The use of humor with children in hospital settings. In P. E. McGhee (ed.), *Humor and children's development:* A guide to practical applications (pp. 157-169). New York: Haworth Press.

Darwin, C. (1872/1965). *The expression of the emotions in man and animals*. Chicago: University of Chicago Press.

de Gaines, P. (1988). *Some days I have cancer more than other days*. Chemo Comics I, P. O. Box 5927, Reno, Nevada 89513.

Deloria, V., Jr. (1969). Indian humor. *Custer died for your sins*. New York: Macmillan.

Dillon, J., & Minchoff, B. (1985-6). Positive emotional states and enhancement of the immune system, *International Journal of Psychiatry in Medicine*, *15* (1), 13-18.

Dobree, B. (1962). Restoration comedy, drama and values. In Felheim, M. (ed.), *Comedy: Plays, Theory and Criticism* (pp. 202-205). New York: Harcourt, Brace and World.

Duchowny, M. S. (1983). Pathological disorders of laughter, In P. E. McGhee & J. H. Goldstein (eds.), *Handbook of Humor Research*, Vol. II, Applied Studies (pp. 87-108). New York: Springer-Verlag.

Dundes, A. (1987). *Cracking jokes*. Studies of sick humor cycles and stereotypes. Berkeley, CA: Ten Speed Press.

Eastman, M. (1921). *The sense of humor*. New York: Schribner.

Eastman, M. (1936). *The enjoyment of laughter*. New York: Simon and Schuster.

Eberhart, E. T. (1988). Humor: hoping and coping. In L. F. Nilsen & A. P. Nilson (eds.), *Whimsy VI, International Humor*, (pp. 265-266). Proceedings of the 6th (1987) Conference. Tempe: Arizona State University.

Eble, K. (1966). *A perfect education*. New York: Macmillan.

Ellis, A. (1987). The use of rational humorous songs in psychotherapy. In W. F. Fry, Jr. & W. A. Salameh (eds.), *Handbook of Humor and Psychotherapy*, (pp. 265-286). Sarasota, FL: Professional Resource Exchange.

Emerson, J. P. (1963). *Social functions of humor in a hospital setting.* Unpublished Ph.D. dissertation, University of California.

Emerson, J. P. (1969). Negotiating the serious import of humor. *Sociometry, 32*, 169-181.

Enck, J. J., Forter, E. T., Whitley, A. (eds.) (1960). *The Comic in Theory and Practice*. New York: Appleton-Century-Crofts.

Esar, E. (1983). *Esar's comic dictionary*. Fourth edition. New York: Doubleday.

Farrelly, F., & Brandsma, J. (1974). *Provocative therapy*. Cupertino, CA: Meta.

Farrelly, F. & Lynch, M. (1987). Humor in Provocative Therapy. In W.F. Fry, Jr. & W.A. Salameh, (eds.) *Handbook of Humor and Psychotherapy*. Advances in clinical use of humor, (pp.81-106). Sarasota, FL: Professional Resource Exchange.

Felheim, M. (1962). *Comedy: plays, theory, and criticism*. New York: Harcourt, Brace and World.

Fine, G. A. (1983). Sociological approaches to the study of humor. In P. E. McGhee & J. H. Goldstein (eds.), *Handbook of humor research: Vol. 1, Basic Issues* (pp. 159-181). New York: Springer-Verlag.

Fisher, S., & Fisher, R. L. (1983). Personality and psychopathology in the comic. In P. E. McGhee & J. H. Goldstein (eds.), *Handbook of humor research: Vol. 2, Applied Studies* (pp. 41-59). New York: Springer-Verlag.

Flugel, J. C. (1954). Humor and laughter. In Lindsay, G. (ed.), *Handbook of Social Psychology* (pp. 709-734). Cambridge, MA: Addison-Wesley.

Foster, H. L. (1974). *Ribbin, jivin', and playin' the dozens: the unrecognized dilemma of inner city schools*. Cambridge, MA: Ballinger Publishing.

Fox, R. C. (1959). *Experiment Perilous*. Glencoe, IL: The Free Press, A. Corporation.

Frankl, V. (1963). *Man's search for meaning*. New York: Washington Square Press.

Freud, S. (1905/1961). *Jokes and their relation to the unconscious*. In Strachey, J. (ed.), *The complete psychological works of Sigmund Freud*, Vol. VIII. London: Hogarth Press.

Freud, S. (1927/1961). Humour. In Strachey, J. (ed.), *The Complete Psychological Works of Sigmund Freud*, Vol. XXI. London: Hogarth Press.

Frey, W. H., II (1985). *Crying: the mystery of tears*. Minneapolis: Winston Press.

Friedman, L. A. (1963). Use of comic effect for control of dysfunctional human behavior in outer space. *Human Factors*, *5*, 355-362.

Frost, R. (1962). Forgive, O Lord. *In the clearing*. New York: Holt, Rinehart and Winston.

Fry, W. F., Jr. (1963). *Sweet Madness:* A study of humor. Palo Alto, CA: Pacific Books.

Fry, W. F., Jr. (1977, a). The appeasement function of mirthful laughter. In A. J. Chapman & H. C. Foot (eds.), *It's a funny thing, humour*, (pp. 23-26). Oxford: Pergamon.

Fry, W. F., Jr. (1977, b). The respiratory components of mirthful laughter. *Journal of Biological Psychology*, *19* (2), 39-50.

Fry, W. F., Jr. (1979). Humor and the human cardiovascular system. In H. Mindess & J. Turek (eds.), *The study of humor*. Los Angeles: Antioch University.

Fry, W. F., Jr. (1986). Humor, physiology, and the aging process. In L. Nahemow, K. A. McCluskey-Fawcett, P. E. McGhee (eds.), *Humor and aging* (pp. 81-98). New York: Academic Press.

Fry, W. F., Jr., & Allen, M. (1975). *Make 'em Laugh: Life studies of comedy writers*. Palo Alto: Science and Behavior Books.

Fry, W. F., Jr., & Salameh, W. A. (eds.) (1987). *Handbook of humor and psychotherapy: advances in the clinical use of humor*. Sarasota, FL: Professional Resource Exchange.

Fry, W. F., Jr., & Savin, M. (1982). *Mirthful laughter and blood pressure*. Paper presented at the Third International Conference on Humor, Washington, DC.

Fry, W. F., Jr., & Stoft, P. E. (1971). Mirth and oxygen saturation levels of peripheral blood. *Psychotherapy and Psychosomatics*, *19*, 76-84.

Gardner, H. (1981). February. How the split brain gets a joke. *Psychology Today*, 74-79.

Gardner, H., Brownell, H.H., Michel, D. & Powelson, J. (1983). Surprise but not coherence: Sensitivity to verbal humor in Right hemisphere patients. *Brain and Language*, *18*, 20-27.

Godkewitsch, M. (1976). Physiological and verbal indices of arousal in rated humor. In A. J. Chapman & H. C. Foot (eds.), *Humour and laughter: Theory, research, and appliances*. (pp. 117-138). London: Wiley.

Goldstein, J. H. (1970). Humor and time to respond. *Psychological Reports*, *27*, 445-446.

Goldstein, J. H. (1987). Therapeutic effects of laughter. In W. F. Fry, Jr., & W. A. Salameh (eds.), *Handbook of humor and psychotherapy*, advances in the clinical use of humor (pp. 1-19). Sarasota, FL: Professional Resource Exchange.

Goldstein, J. H., McGhee, P. E. (1972). *The psychology of humor*. Theoretical perspectives and empirical issues. New York: Academic Press.

Goodman, J. (1983). How to get more smileage out of your life. In P. E. McGhee & J. H. Goldstein (eds.), *Handbook of Humor Research*, Volume II, Applied Studies (pp. 1-21). New York: Springer-Verlag.

Goodman, J. (1989). A real jewell. *Laughing Matters*, 5(3), 87-99.

Goodrich, A. T., Jules, H., Goodrich, D. W. (1954). Laughter in psychiatric staff conferences: a sociopsychiatric analysis. *American Journal of Orthopsychiatry*, *24*, 175-184.

Greenwald, H. (1973). *Direct decision therapy*. San Diego, CA: EDITS.

Greenwald, H. (1987). The humor decision. In W. F. Fry, Jr., & W. A. Salameh (eds.), *Handbook of humor and psychotherapy* (p. 41-54). Sarasota, FL: Professional Resource Exchange.

Grotjahn, M. (1957). *Beyond laughter*. New York: The Blakiston Division, McGraw-Hill.

Hageseth, C. (1988). *A laughing place*. Fort Collins, CO: Berwick Publishing.

Haig, R. A. (1988). *The anatomy of humor: Biopsychosocial and therapeutic perspectives*. Springfield, IL: Charles C. Thomas.

Harrel, S. (1962). *When it's laughter you're after*. Norman, OK: University of Oklahoma Press.

Hayworth, D. (1928). The social origins and functions of laughter. *Psychological Review*, *35*, 367-384.

Hazlitt, W. (1819/1960). Lecture on Wit and Humor. In Enck, J.J., Forter, E. T., & Witley, A. (eds.), *The comic in theory and practice* (pp. 16-21). New York: Appleton- Century-Crofts.

Helitzer, M. (1984). *Comedy: Techniques for writers and performers*. Athens, OH: Lawford Press.

Heller, J. (1955). *Catch 22*. New York: Dell Publishing.

Herth, K. (1984). Laughter: A nursing RX. *American Journal of Nursing*, *84*(8), 991-992.

Hill, H. (1968). Black humor: its cause and cure. *Colorado Quarterly* XVII pp. 57-64.

Hill, W. (1943). *Navajo Humor*. Menasha: Banta.

Hines, R. H. (1972). Health status of black Americans. In Jaco, G. E. (ed.), *Patients, physicians and illness*, 2nd ed. (pp. 40-50). New York: Free Press.

Hobbes, T. (1650/1987). Human nature. In J. Morreall (ed.), *The philosophy of laughter and humor* (pp. 19-20). Albany: State University of New York Press.

Isen, A. M., Daubman, K. A., Nowicki, G. P. (1987). Positive affect facilitates creative problem solving. *Journal of Personality and Social Psychology*, *52*, (6) 1122-1131.

Jackson, M. (1985). The comedy of management. In L. Simms, S. Price & N. Ervin, *The Professional Practice of Nursing Administration*, (pp. 339-351). New York: Wiley.

Jaeger, D. & Simmons, L. W. (1970). *The aged ill* Coping with problems in geriatric care. New York: Appleton-Century- Crofts.

Johnston, W. (1985). To the one's left behind. *American Journal of Nursing*, *85* (8), 936.

Kanin, C. (1978). *It takes a long time to become young.* New York: Doubleday.

Kant, I. (1790/1987). Critique of judgment. In J. Morreall (ed.), *The philosophy of laughter and humor* (pp. 45-50). Albany: State University of New York Press.

Kaplan, H., & Boyd, I. H. (1965). The social functions of humor on an open psychiatric ward. *Psychiatric Quarterly*, *39*, 502-515.

Kaufman, G. & Blakely, M. K. (eds.) (1980). *Pulling our own strings*: Feminist humor and satire. Bloomington: Indiana University Press.

Keith-Spiegel, P. (1972). Early conceptions of humor: Varieties and issues. In J. H. Goldstein & P. E. McGhee (eds.), *The psychology of humor*, (pp. 3-39). New York: Academic Press.

Kesey, K. (1962). *One flew over the cuckoo's nest.* New York: Signet Books.

Kevin, Sister M. (1964). How to recognize your patient's humors. *RN*, December (51-53).

Klapp, O. (1950). The fool as a social type. *American Journal of Sociology*, *55*, 157-162.

Klein, A. (1989). *The healing power of humor.* Techniques for getting through loss, setbacks, upsets, disappointments, difficulties, trials, tribulations, and all that not-so-funny stuff. Los Angeles: J. P. Tarcher.

Kluckhohn, C., & Leighton, D. C. (1946). *The Navajo.* Cambridge: Harvard University Press.

Koestler, A. (1964). *The act of creation.* New York: Macmillan.

Kronenberger, L. (1952). *The thread of laughter.* New York: Alfred A. Knopf.

Kubie, L. S. (1971). The destructive potential of humor in psychotherapy. *American Journal of Psychiatry, 127,* 861-866.

Kuhlman, T. L. (1984). *Humor and psychotherapy.* Homewood, IL: Dow Jones-Irwin.

Landon, M. D. (1883). *Wit and humor of the age.* Chicago: Star Publishing.

Langevin, R., & Day, H. I. (1972). Physiological correlates of humor. In J. H. Goldstein & P. E. McGhee (eds.), *The psychology of humor,* (pp. 129-142). New York: Academic Press.

Lazarus, R. S., & Folkman, S. (1984). *Stress, appraisal and coping.* New York: Springer.

Lefrancois, G. R. (1972). *Psychological theories and human learning: Kongor's report.* Monterey, CA: Brooks-Cole Publishing.

Leiber, D. B. (1986). Laughter and humor in critical care. *Dimensions of critical care nursing. 5* (3), 162-170.

Leighton, A., & Leighton, D. C. (1944). *The Navajo door.* Cambridge, MA: Harvard Press.

Leininger, M. (1970). *Nursing and anthropology: Two worlds to blend.* New York: John Wiley and Sons.

Levine, J. (1956). Responses to humor. *Scientific American, 194,* (212), 31-35.

Levine, J. (1961). Regression in primitive clowning. *Psychoanalytic Quarterly 30,* 72-83.

Levine, J. (1968). Humor. *International encyclopedia of the social sciences,* VII, 1-7, David Sills (ed.). New York: Macmillan.

Levine, J., & Redlich, F. (1955). Failure to understand humor. *Psychoanalytic Quarterly 24,* 560-572.

Long, P. (1987). Laugh and be well? *Psychology Today, 21* 10, 28-29.

Lorenz, K. (1963). *On aggression.* New York: Harcourt, Brace and World.

Madanes, C. (1987). Humor in strategic family therapy. In W. F. Fry, Jr. & W. A. Salameh (eds.), *Handbook of humor and psychotherapy* (pp. 241-264). Sarasota, FL: Professional Resource Exchange.

Madsen, W. (1964). *The Mexican-Americans of South Texas.* New York: Holt, Rinehart and Winston.

Martin, R. A. (1989). Humor and mastery of living: Using humor to cope with the daily stresses of growing up. In P. E. McGhee (ed.), *Humor and children's development: a guide to practical applications* (pp. 135-155), New York: Haworth.

Maslow, A. H. (1970). *Motivation and personality,* 2nd ed. New York: Harper and Row.

McCabe, G. S. (1960). Cultural influences on patient behavior. *The American Journal of Nursing, 60* (8), 1101-1104.

McDougall, W. (1963). An instinct of laughter. *An introduction to social psychology*. New York: University Paperbacks, Barnes and Noble.

McGhee, P. E. (1979). *Humor: Origins and development*. San Francisco: Freeman.

McGhee, P. E. (ed.) (1989). *Humor and children's development: a guide to practical applications*. New York: Haworth.

McGhee, P. E., & Chapman, A. J. (eds.) (1980). *Children's humour*, Chichester, England: Wiley.

McGhee, P. E., & Goldstein, J. H. (eds.) (1983). *Handbook of humor research: Volume I, Basic Issues; Volume II, Applied Studies*. New York: Springer-Verlag.

McLuhan, M. (1967). *The medium is the massage*. New York: Bantam Books.

Meeker, J. W. (1972). *The comedy of survival: studies in literary ecology*. New York: Charles Scribner's Sons.

Mendel, W. (ed.) (1970). *A celebration of laughter*. Los Angeles: Mara Books.

Meredith, G. (1877/1962). Lecture: On comedy and the uses of the comic spirit. In M. Felheim (ed.), *Comedy: plays, theory, and criticism* (pp. 205-214). New York: Harcourt, Brace and World.

Middleton, R., & Moland, J. (1959). Humor in negro and white subcultures: a study of jokes among university students. *American Sociological Review* 24, 61-69.

Mikes, G. (1971). *Laughing matter*. New York: The Library Press.

Mindess, H. (1971). *Laughter and liberation*. Los Angeles: Nash Publishing Company.

Mindess, H. (1976). The use and abuse of humour in psychotherapy. In A. J. Chapman & H. C. Foot (eds.), *Humour and laughter: Theory, research, and applications*. (pp. 331-341). London: Wiley.

Mindess, H., Miller, C., Turek, J., Bender, A., & Corbin, S. (1985). *The Antioch humor test: making sense of humor*. New York: Argon Books.

Monro, D. H. (1951). *Argument of laughter*. Melbourne: Melbourne University Press.

Moody, R. A. (1978). *Laugh after laugh*. Jacksonville, FL: Headwaters Press.

Morreall, J. (1983). *Taking laughter seriously*. Albany: State University of New York Press.

Morreall, J. (ed.) (1987). *The philosophy of laughter and humor*. Albany: State University of New York Press.

Mintz, L. E. (ed.) (1988). *Humor in America*. A research guide to genres and topics. Westport, CT: Greenwood.

Murphy, B., & Pollio, H. R. (1973). I'll laugh if you will. *Psychology Today*, December, 106-109.

Myrdal, G. (1944). *An American dilemma*. New York: Harper.

Naisbett, J. (1982). *Megatrends: Ten new directions transforming our lives*. New York: Warner Books.

Nava, J. (1971). Foreword. In Wagner, N. N., Haug, M. J. (eds.), *Chicanos: social and psychological perspectives* (pp. xxi-xxiii). Saint Louis: C. V. Mosby.

Nilsen, D. L. F., Nilsen, A. P., with K. Donelson (1988). Humor in the United States. In A. Ziv (ed.), *National styles of humor* (pp. 157-158). Westport, CT: Greenwood.

Norris, C. (1961-62). Greetings from a lonely crowd. *Nursing Forum, 1*, 73-82).

Nussbaum, K., & Michaux, W. W. (1963). Response to humor in depression: a predictor and evaluator of patient change. *Psychiatric Quarterly 37*, 527-539.

Obrdlik, A. J. (1942). Gallows humor -- a sociological phenomenon. *American Journal of Sociology 47*, 709-716.

O'Connell, W. E. (1976). Freudian humor: The eupsychia of everyday life. In A. J. Chapman & H. C. Foot (eds.), *Humour and laughter: theory, research, and applications*. (pp. 313-330). London: Wiley.

O'Connell, W. E. (1987). Natural high theory and practice: the humorist's game of games. In W. F. Fry, Jr., & W. A. Salameh (eds.), *Handbook of humor and psychotherapy* (pp. 55- 79). Sarasota, FL: Professional Resource Exchange.

O'Connell, W. E., & Covert, C. (1967). Death attitudes and humor appreciation among medical students. *Existential Psychiatry, 6*, 433-442.

Orben, R. (1963). *If you have to be a comic*. Wilmington, DE: The Comedy Center.

Orben, R. (1972). The Pied Piper of humor. *Talent*, Spring (pp. 34-36). Cleveland, OH: International Platform Association.

Orben, R. (1988). Uses and limits of humor. *Orben's current comedy*. Excerpt in *Humor events and possibilities*. Workshop library on world humor. Non-volume minus thirty- seven, Spring 1989.

Pearson, G. A. (1965). A child's humor. *Nursing Science 3*, 95-108.

Peter, L., & Dana, B. (1982). *The laughter prescription*. New York: Ballantine Books.

Piddington, R. (1933/1963). *The psychology of laughter*. New York: Gamut Press.

Poland, W. S. (1971). The place of humor in psychotherapy. *American Journal of Psychiatry 128*, 635-637.

Powell, B. S. (1974). Laughter and healing: the use of humor in hospitals treating children. *Association for the Care of Children in Hospitals Journal*, November, 10-16.

Radcliffe-Brown, A. R. (1952). On joking relationships. *Structure and function in primitive society*. New York: Free Press.

Rapp, A. (1951). *The origins of wit and humor*. New York: Dutton.

Reese, R. L. (1967). Does humor have a place in scientific writing? *American Medical Writers' Association Bulletin*, *17*, 11-13.

Reichard, G. (1950). *Navajo religion, a study of symbolism*. New York: Bolligen Foundation.

Rivera, M.E. (1988). The magic and power of children's humor. *Child Action News*. Jul/Aug/Sep. p. 4.

Robinson, V. M. (1970/1978). Humor in nursing. In C. Carlson & B. Blackwell (eds.), *Behavioral concepts and nursing intervention*, (pp. 191-210) 2nd ed. Philadelphia: Lippincott.

Robinson, V. M. (1983). Humor and health. In P. E. McGhee & J. H. Goldstein (eds.), *Handbook of humor research*, Volume II, Applied Studies (pp. 109-128). New York: Springer-Verlag.

Robinson, V. M. (1986). Humor is a serious business. (Editorial). *Dimensions of Critical Care Nursing*, *5* (3), 132-33.

Robinson, V. M. (1988). A study of recalled and reported observations of humor in health care settings. In D. Nilsen & A. Nilsen (eds.), *Whimsy VI: International Humor*. (pp. 200-201). Proceedings of 6th Conference. Tempe: Arizona State University.

Rogers, C. (1969). *Freedom to learn*. Columbus, OH: Charles E. Merrill.

Rose, G. J. (1969). King Lear and the use of humor in treatment. *Journal of the American Psychoanalytic Association*, *12*, 927-940.

Salameh, W. A. (1983). Humor in psychotherapy: past outlooks, present status and future frontiers. In P. E. McGhee & J. H. Goldstein (eds.), *Handbook of humor research*, Volume II (pp. 61-88). New York: Springer-Verlag.

Salameh, W. A. (1987). Humor in integrative short-term psychotherapy (ISTP). In W. F. Fry, Jr., & W. A. Salameh (eds.), *Handbook of humor and psychotherapy* (pp. 195-240). Sarasota, FL: Professional Resource Exchange.

Sanders, D. H. (1973). *Computers in society*. New York: McGraw-Hill.

Schachter, S., & Wheeler, L. (1962). Epinephrine, chlorpromazine and amusement. *Journal of Abnormal and Social Psychology*, *65*, 121-128.

Schulz, M. F. (1973). *Black humor fiction in the sixties*. Athens, OH: Ohio University Press.

Siegal, B. S. (1986). *Love, medicine, and miracles*. New York: Harper and Row.

Simmons, D. (1963). Protest humor: Folkloristic reaction to prejudice. *American Journal of Psychiatry, 120*, 567-570.

Simonton, O. C, Matthews-Simonton, S., & Creighton, J. (1978). *Getting well again*. Los Angeles: J. P. Tarcher.

Spencer, H. (1860). The physiology of laughter. *Macmillan's Magazine, 1*, 395-402.

Spitz, R. (1946). The smiling response: a contribution to the ontogenesis of social relations. *Genetic Psychology Monographs, 34*, 57-125.

Steiner, S. (1968). *The new Indians*. New York: Harper and Row.

Stephenson, R. M. (1959). Conflict and control functions of humor. *American Journal of Sociology, 56*, 569-574.

Sully, J. (1902/1963). Essay on laughter. *The psychology of laughter: a study in social adaptation* (pp. 196-200). New York: Gamut Press.

Suls, J. (1983). Cognitive processes in humor appreciation. In P. E. McGhee & J. H. Goldstein (eds.), *Handbook of humor research*, Volume I, Basic Issues (pp. 39-57). New York: Springer-Verlag.

Svebak, S. (1975). Respiratory patterns as predictors of laughter. *Psychophysiology, 12*, 62-65.

Svebak, S. (1977). Some characteristics of resting respiration as predictors of laughter: In A. J. Chapman & H. C. Foot (eds.), *It's a funny thing, humour*, (pp. 101-104). Oxford: Pergamon.

Svebak, S. (1982). The effect of mirthfulness upon amount of discordant right-left occipital EEG Alpha. *Motivation and emotion, 6*, 133-143.

Thompson, S. (1946). The trickster cycle. *The folktale* (pp. 319-328). New York: Dryden Press.

Valiant, G. E. (1977). *Adaptation to life*. Boston: Little, Brown.

Vargas, M. J. (1961). Uses of humor in group psychotherapy. *Group Psychotherapy, 14*, 198-202.

Ventis, W. L. (1987). Humor and laughter in behavior therapy. In W. F. Fry, Jr., & W. A. Salameh (eds.), *Handbook of humor and psychotherapy* (pp. 149-170). Sarasota, FL: Professional Resource Exchange.

Ventis, W. L., & Ventis, D. G. (1989). Guidelines for using humor in therapy with children and young adolescents. In P. E. McGhee (ed.), *Humor and children's development: a guide to practical applications* (pp. 179-197). New York: Haworth.

Walsh, J. J. (1928). *Laughter and health*. New York: Appleton.

Warner, S. L. (1984). Humor and self-disclosure within the milieu. *Journal of Psychosocial Nursing, 22*(4), 17-21.

Warner, S. L. (1986). Appropriate uses of humor in critical care. *Dimensions of critical care nursing, 5*(3), 168-170.

Watson, M. J., & Emerson, S. (1988). Facilitate learning with humor. *Journal of Nursing Education, 27*(2), 89-90.

Weinstein, M., & Goodman, J. (1986). *Playfair: everybody's guide to non-competitive play*. San Luis Obispo, CA: Impact Publishers.

Wessell, Sister M. L. (1975). Use of humor by an immobilized adolescent girl during hospitalization. *Maternal-Child Nursing Journal, 4*(1), 35-48.

White, E. B. (1954/1960). Some remarks on humor. The second tree from the corner. New York: Harper and Brothers. In Enck, J. J., Forter, E. T., & Whitley, A. (eds.), *The comic in theory and practice* (pp. 102-108). New York: Appleton- Century-Crofts.

Whiting, P. (1969). *How to speak and write with humor*. New York: McGraw-Hill.

Wolfenstein, M. (1954). *Children's humor*. Glencoe, IL: Free Press.

Zillman, D., & Bryant, J. (1983). Uses and effects of humor in educational ventures. In P. E. McGhee & J. H. Goldstein (eds.), *Handbook of humor research*, Volume II, Applied Studies (pp. 173-193). New York: Springer-Verlag.

Ziv, A. (1976). The effects of humor in creativity. *Journal of Educational Psychology, 3*, 318-322.

Ziv, A. (1979). The teacher's sense of humour and the atmosphere in the classroom. *School Psychology International*, September/October, 21-23.

Ziv, A. (1980). Humor and creativity. *The Creative Child and Adult Quarterly, 5*(3), 159-170.

Ziv, A. (1981). The self concept of adolescent humorists. *Journal of Adolescence, 4*, 187-197.

Ziv, A. (1983). The influence of humorous atmosphere on divergent thinking. *Contemporary Educational Psychology, 8*, 413-421.

Ziv, A. (1984). *Personality and sense of humor*. New York: Springer.

Ziv, A. (ed.) (1988). *National styles of humor*. Westport, CT: Greenwood.

Ziv, A. (1989). Using humor to develop creative thinking. In P. E. McGhee, (ed.), *Humor and children's development: a guide to practical applications*. New York: Haworth.

Zolten, J. J. (1988). Humor and the Challenger shuttle disaster: joke-telling as a reaction to tragedy. In D. Nilsen & A. Nilsen (eds.), *Whimsy VI: International Humor* Proceedings of 6th Conference (pp. 134-136). Tempe: Arizona State University.

Zwerling, I. (1955). The favorite joke in diagnostic and therapeutic interviewing. *Psychoanalytic Quarterly, 24*, 104-114.

# Index